He kept the conversation light all the way to her house. "See you at work on Monday."

He kissed her lingeringly, and even though it was still raining, his kiss made her feel as if it was the middle of the day, with the sun shining brightly. How was it that he could make her feel that kind of warmth, that kind of brightness?

"Monday," she said and kissed him one last time before climbing out of the car. She turned to wave at him just before she opened her front door, and he blew her a kiss.

Cute.

Nathaniel Jones was seriously cute.

And she was going to have to be careful, or she'd be in danger of losing her heart to him completely.

Dear Reader,

I read a couple of articles that fascinated me—one about the fact there are only a couple of hundred male midwives in the UK, and one about a man whose life-changing accident made him switch careers to nursing. And that started me thinking about writing a book about a male midwife and a female obstetrician. What happens when you have two people who've been through a lot come out the other side and are scared to trust again in case it goes wrong? How do they learn to trust their own judgments, as well as each other?

I hope you enjoy Rebecca and Nathaniel's story.

With love,

Kate Hardy

FOREVER FAMILY FOR THE MIDWIFE

KATE HARDY

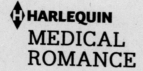

HARLEQUIN
MEDICAL
ROMANCE

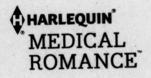

Recycling programs for this product may not exist in your area.

ISBN-13: 978-1-335-14983-1

Forever Family for the Midwife

This edition published by arrangement with Harlequin Books S.A.

For questions and comments about the quality of this book, please contact us at CustomerService@Harlequin.com.

Harlequin Enterprises ULC
22 Adelaide St. West, 40th Floor
Toronto, Ontario M5H 4E3, Canada
www.Harlequin.com

Printed in U.S.A.

Kate Hardy has always loved books and could read before she went to school. She discovered Harlequin books when she was twelve and decided that this was what she wanted to do. When she isn't writing, Kate enjoys reading, cinema, ballroom dancing and the gym. You can contact her via her website: katehardy.com.

Books by Kate Hardy

Harlequin Medical Romance

Changing Shifts
Fling with Her Hot-Shot Consultant

Miracles at Muswell Hill Hospital
Christmas with Her Daredevil Doc
Their Pregnancy Gift

Unlocking the Italian Doc's Heart
Carrying the Single Dad's Baby
Heart Surgeon, Prince…Husband!
A Nurse and a Pup to Heal Him
Mistletoe Proposal on the Children's Ward

Harlequin Romance

A Crown by Christmas
Soldier Prince's Secret Baby Gift

A Diamond in the Snow
Finding Mr. Right in Florence
One Night to Remember
A Will, a Wish, a Wedding

Visit the Author Profile page
at Harlequin.com for more titles.

To Julia Williams and Chere Tricot, with love
and thanks for their patience and kindness when
lockdown made writing very difficult! xxx

CHAPTER ONE

'I'M NOT HAVING you touching my wife.'

The words were audible right across the ward.

The raised voices weren't just going to upset the poor mum-to-be in that room, they were going to upset all the other mums-to-be within earshot. And none of them needed the extra stress during labour. Rebecca knew that the head of midwifery was in a meeting with the consultants, so she was probably the most senior person on the ward at that moment—meaning that she was the one who needed to deal with this. She walked swiftly over to the room, preparing to calm everything down.

'Everything all right?' she asked sweetly, knowing perfectly well that it wasn't, but also knowing that going in and shouting just as loudly wasn't going to help anyone.

'No, it isn't.' A stocky man stood in front of

the bed with his fists clenched. 'I'm not having *him* touching my wife.'

'Him' being the midwife. Rebecca hadn't met Nathaniel Jones yet, as she'd been on leave for the last two weeks since he'd joined the maternity team at Muswell Hill Memorial Hospital, but she knew he was one of the very few male midwives in the country. And this situation needed to be de-escalated as fast as possible.

'Let me introduce myself,' Rebecca said. 'I'm Dr Hart, obstetric registrar. Why don't you come over to my office, where it's a bit more private, and we can discuss it?'

'What, and leave *him* here with my wife?' the man demanded.

'Mr—' This couple hadn't been to any of her clinics, and one of her colleagues had done the ward round this morning, so she didn't know their names. She glanced at the whiteboard above the bed, where the words 'Ruth Brown' had been written, and hoped that her assumption wouldn't make things worse. 'Mr Brown. Your wife's on our ward right now, and our priority is to keep her comfortable and the baby safe,' she said calmly.

'I'm fully qualified,' Nathaniel said gently, 'and Dr Hart is right—your wife and baby are our priorities. Just to reassure you, I had to deliver forty babies before I could qualify, and I've delivered a few more since then. Your wife is very safe with me—my job is to listen to her and help.'

'It's not that. I'm not having a man looking at her...' Mr Brown gave a jerk of his head. 'Down there.'

Oh, for pity's sake. This was a maternity unit! But she bit back her impatience; telling the man he was being an idiot would only put his back up even more and make things worse. 'While you and I have a chat, are you OK for Mr Jones to take your wife's temperature, blood pressure and pulse rate, and keep a check on the baby's movements?'

'I suppose so,' Mr Brown admitted grudgingly.

'Good. Let's go to my office,' she said, giving Nathaniel a reassuring smile. 'We'll be back in a minute, Mrs Brown.' She led Mr Brown to her office and closed the door to give them privacy.

Clearly she'd meant well, but Nathaniel was a little bit irritated that Rebecca Hart had swept in to deal with a situation he was perfectly capable of handling himself. He really hoped she wasn't the sort of doctor who felt the need to pull rank on a midwife; he'd worked with that sort before and in his view the mum's needs should come before everything else. Or was she like one of his tutors, feeling that men had no place as a midwife?

He took a deep breath to stem his irritation and turned to Ruth Brown. 'Mrs Brown, I'm sorry about that,' he said.

She grimaced. 'I should be the one apologising. Mike was so rude to you.'

'Hey. That's not important. *You* are,' he said. 'And I'm guessing your blood pressure isn't going to be great, so either I can regale you with some terrible jokes or you can do some breathing exercises to help you relax a bit before I put the cuff on your arm.'

As he'd hoped, she laughed and looked less awkward. 'I'll do the breathing. Mike doesn't mean to be rude. We had a scare a couple of weeks back, when I couldn't feel the baby moving. And he's a typical bloke—can't say what he feels, so he gets cross instead. Oh, present company excepted,' she added.

Nathaniel laughed. 'Fair point, and I don't think I'm an exception. I don't know many men who are good at talking about their feelings. Right. Let's try that blood pressure…'

'I've never heard of a bloke being a midwife,' Mr Brown said, his mouth twisted into a sneer.

'What's he doing it for—so he can look at women down there?'

'No. There are several hundred male midwives across the country, and they do it for exactly the same reason our female midwives do their job—the same reason that I, as a senior doctor, do my job. To deliver babies safely,' Rebecca said, keeping her voice cool and even.

'It's not *right*, a bloke being a midwife,' Mr Brown continued, his face flushed with anger.

'Nathaniel is qualified and he's experienced,' Rebecca said. 'If I was in labour, I'd want someone like him to look after me. A trained midwife, who'd be able to spot the signs of any problem right in the early stages and could sort it out before it became an emergency.'

'I suppose,' Mr Brown acknowledged. 'But I still don't want him looking after my wife.'

'Would you have a problem with your wife being seen by a male doctor?' she asked.

He looked surprised. 'Well, no.'

'It's the same thing,' she pointed out gently. 'Just a different title.'

He shook his head. 'Midwives aren't doctors.'

Midwives were just as important as doctors, but this wasn't the right time to have that argument. She needed to deal with the immediate situation first. 'I can talk to the midwifery team to see if anyone else is available to look after your wife,' she said. 'But I can't guarantee there will be.' She could see fear in Mr Brown's face. Was it fear that was driving all this? 'Is this your first baby?' she asked gently.

He nodded.

'It's exciting, because you can't wait to meet your baby, the one you've felt kick and seen on a scan; but it's also really scary, because you see all these awful things on the internet. All the horror stories of things going wrong.' She'd just bet Mr Brown was familiar with 'Dr Search Engine'—and she really hoped that he hadn't seen fit to share his findings with his wife.

'Yeah,' he admitted. 'Ruth couldn't feel the baby moving, a couple of weeks back. I drove her here so fast I got stopped by the police. But when I told them why, they escorted us in with their blue lights going.'

'And everything was all right?' Well, obviously, or she wouldn't be in labour. But he was talking now and Rebecca wanted to keep that going.

'We had a scan and the baby was kicking.' A muscle tensed in his jaw. 'But the doctors said the baby's a bit small for dates. That's why they wanted Ruth to come in today and be induced.'

'So you came in first thing this morning?'

He nodded. 'We had a different midwife

when we came in. She said she was going to do this membrane sweep thing.'

'That's an internal exam, which separates the membranes of the fluid-filled sac around the baby from the cervix, releasing the hormones that kick-start labour,' Rebecca said, sure that the midwife had already explained the process but wanting to make completely certain that Mr Brown understood what was happening. 'I assume her labour hasn't started yet?'

'No. And *he* said he'd insert a pessary. In her...' He paused, looking embarrassed and cross.

'Your first midwife probably—' *definitely* '—told you that might need to happen if Ruth's contractions hadn't started within six hours,' she said gently.

'I didn't really take it all in,' Mr Brown admitted. 'I was just worried about Ruthie and the baby.'

'OK. When we induce labour, if the membrane sweep doesn't work then we'll insert a tablet of the prostaglandin hormones into the vagina.' Rebecca chose her words carefully, keeping everything as impersonal and cool as possible. 'Sometimes it takes a second tablet before labour actually starts. Right now, I think you need someone experienced looking after your wife. Someone who understands about the scare you had during pregnancy, and how worrying it is to have your labour started for you instead of it all happening naturally. You need someone who's going to keep a really good eye on your wife and the baby. Someone who sees her as a mum-to-be and understands her worries—and yours, too. If anything, I reckon Mr Jones is going to be able to help you a bit more than a female midwife could because he'll have a better idea of what goes through a bloke's head.'

Mr Brown shuffled in his chair.

Clearly he was still focusing on the idea of another man looking at and touching his wife's vagina. So she was going to have to embarrass him slightly. 'I can assure you, Mr Jones won't be looking at your wife in the same way you do,' she said, as kindly as she could. 'Just as if, say, you had a lump in your testicles and I was your GP and needed to examine you.'

This time, his face went a very deep shade of crimson.

'I'd examine you, because that's my job,' she said, 'but I wouldn't be looking at your body in the same way that your wife does. I'd see you as my patient—someone who's worried, who has a symptom on a part of his body and who needs my help. There wouldn't be anything at all sexual in the way I looked at you, just as there's nothing sexual in the way Mr Jones looks at your wife. He'll simply be following the procedures, just as a female midwife would.'

'I guess,' Mr Brown said.

'If a female midwife isn't available and you're really concerned about the propriety of having a male midwife, we can arrange for a chaperone,' she said. He'd said earlier that he wouldn't object to a male doctor, so maybe this was the best way to make the point. 'And if any of our male doctors need to see her, we can also arrange for a chaperone for them if that would make you feel more comfortable.'

She waited for him to think about it.

Eventually he looked at her. 'I'm making a fuss over nothing, aren't I?' he asked.

'You're worried about your wife and the baby,' she said. 'But you're also worrying about something that isn't an issue, so that's one burden you can choose to take off your shoulders and make your life a bit easier.'

He took a deep breath. 'All right. He can do it.'

'Thank you.'

'And we don't need a chaperone.'

Relief flooded through her. She smiled. 'Rest assured, all the staff here will treat your wife— and you—with the utmost dignity and respect.

But I'd also like to remind you, Mr Brown, that the hospital has a zero-tolerance policy. Our staff have the right to care for our mums-to-be without being attacked or abused, physically or verbally.'

He shuffled in the chair again. 'I owe that bloke an apology, don't I?'

Yes, he did. 'That's your call,' she said, still keeping things calm.

'I'm sorry. I just—I panic, sometimes. I'm used to...' His voice tailed off.

Used to blustering and shouting at his juniors at work if things didn't go quite according to plan? She knew the type. But this wasn't a battle worth fighting. She'd dealt with the important bit so Mrs Brown would get the care she needed. 'OK. Shall we go back and see how your wife's doing?'

He looked shamefaced. 'Ruth's going to kill me.'

'As she's being induced, I think she might have something else distracting her,' Rebecca said with a smile. Mr Brown needed distracting, too, given an important job to stop him overthinking things and getting upset and shouty again. 'And I'm pretty sure she'd like you to do some hand-holding. To chat to her and keep her mind off the wait, because this bit of an induced birth can really get boring. She'll need you to rub her back when she's having a contraction, or get her some really cold water, or fetch her a sandwich when she's getting hungry—that sort of thing.'

'Yeah, I suppose.'

'Shall we go back?'

He nodded.

She escorted him back to the ward where Mrs Brown was waiting on the bed with Nathaniel sitting on the chair next to her, the curtains drawn round them. She was chatting to Nathaniel, clearly completely at ease with him.

Mr Brown walked over to the bed. 'Sorry, mate. I was in the wrong,' he muttered, holding his hand out to shake Nathaniel's.

'You're all right,' Nathaniel said, shaking his hand. 'First babies can do that to you, especially when you've already had a scare and your wife's being induced, and you feel a bit helpless because she's the one going through it and you're not really sure what you can do to make things better.'

Clearly Mrs Brown had filled him in on the situation, Rebecca thought. And Nathaniel was handling this brilliantly, empathising with a scared dad-to-be.

'Yeah,' Mr Brown said.

'You're such an idiot, Mike. Nathaniel's been really good,' Mrs Brown said. 'So are you going to stop making a fuss now and let us get on with having this baby?'

Mr Brown nodded, looking hangdog.

'You could go and get your wife a cup of tea while I sort out the prostaglandin,' Nathaniel suggested, clearly sensitive to what one of the big problems had been.

'I will,' Mr Brown said. 'Can I get anything for you?'

Nathaniel smiled. 'I'm fine, but thanks for asking.'

'I'd like a chicken salad sandwich on whole-meal with that cup of tea, please, love. I'm starving,' Mrs Brown added.

When Mr Brown had left, Mrs Brown said, 'Mike doesn't mean to be an idiot. He's just...' She wrinkled her nose. 'A bit old-school, I suppose.'

'I've reassured him,' Rebecca said. 'I think he realises now that medics don't see their patients in a sexual way, so he won't worry any more.'

Mrs Brown rolled her eyes. 'Open up, ground, and swallow me now,' she said. 'I'm so sorry.'

'There's no need to apologise. A lot of dads-to-be feel like that, at first. It's all fine. Let's concentrate on you and the baby,' Nathaniel said. 'Now, let's get you comfortable and see if we can get this labour up and running.'

'I'm going to back to my paperwork before my clinic. Call me if you need anything,' Rebecca said.

'Thank you,' he said, though there was something in his eyes that said he had no intention of calling her. She suppressed a sigh; the last thing she needed was a team member with a chip on his shoulder. There wasn't room for egos in this job. Their mums-to-be and babies always came first.

The afternoon ward rounds and clinic took up most of the rest of her day. She was just finishing some paperwork when there was a knock on her open door. She looked up to see Nathaniel standing there.

'Dr Hart.'

Normally she would've suggested first-name terms and asked how he was settling in to the team, but his attitude earlier had irritated her. 'Yes, Mr Jones?'

'I thought you'd like to know that the Browns had a healthy little girl, two point six kilos.'

'That's great news,' she said, pleased. 'Thanks for telling me.'

He smiled. 'They both want her middle name to be Natalie, after me.'

Only a few hours ago, Mr Brown had been

yelling that he didn't want Nathaniel anywhere near his wife, and now he wanted to call his daughter after their male midwife?

And then it hit her: she'd steamed in and assumed he needed help to defuse the situation. He could've done it perfectly well himself.

'I'm sorry,' she said.

He frowned. 'Why?'

'When I came in earlier, during the shouty bit. Of course you could handle things.'

He smiled at her, then, and a tingle ran down her spine. A tingle she suppressed ruthlessly; even if he wasn't involved elsewhere, as a single mum she wasn't interested in dating.

'Mike Brown *was* disturbing the ward. I can see where you were coming from,' he said.

'All the same, I think we might have got off on the wrong foot.'

He gave her an assessing look. 'You must be due a break. Let me buy you a coffee.'

'Thanks for offering,' she said, 'but there's really no need. We're a team on this ward and we support each other.'

'All my midwife colleagues are either with a mum or they've finished their shift and gone home. I've just delivered a baby and right now I really want to babble about how amazing it is, to someone who actually gets it.'

'And I'm the only one around?'

'Pretty much.' He gave her another of those smiles that made her stomach swoop, and it unsettled her. She wasn't used to reacting like this to someone.

'Coffee and cake. My shout. And you can let me babble about babies.' He gave her another of those incredibly winning smiles.

Part of her resisted. This man was charming—and she knew from personal experience that charming was fun for a while and then slid into heartbreak. On the other hand, he was her new colleague, they'd started off on the wrong foot and she wanted to smooth things over between them. 'OK, but only if I buy.'

'Dr Hart, it's coffee. No strings,' he said gently.

Which made her face feel hot with embarrassment. 'Sorry,' she mumbled.

'By the way, what did you say to Mike Brown?' he asked, sounding curious.

'I pointed out that if I was a GP looking at a lump on his testicle, I'd see him as a worried patient, not a sex object, and you wouldn't be leering at the business end of his wife because your job was to deliver the baby safely and make sure she was OK during labour. Or something along those lines.'

He grinned, his dark eyes crinkling at the corners, and Rebecca noticed how long his eyelashes were. 'I wish I'd seen his face when you said that.'

'Patient confidentiality,' Rebecca said, knowing how prim she sounded but unable to stop it.

'He really squirmed, didn't he?' His grin broadened. 'To be fair, I would've squirmed, too. Let's go get that coffee.'

She saved the file, logged out of the computer system and walked with him to the canteen.

'How do you like it?' he asked.

Coffee. He was talking about *coffee*. For pity's sake, why was she reacting to him like this? She never flirted. Not since Lucas. And she wasn't going to start flirting now. 'Skinny cappuccino, no chocolate on top, please.'

'OK. Cake?'

'I'm not really a cake person,' she said. 'Though thanks for the offer.'

'Something savoury?'

'Just coffee's lovely, thanks.'

Once he'd ordered their coffee—and cake for himself—they found a quiet table.

'I was away when you joined the team. How are you settling in?' Rebecca asked.

'Pretty good—the staff are all lovely, here,' Nathaniel said. 'I trained at the London Victoria, but I've always liked this part of the city, so when the job came up I applied for it.' He paused. 'How about you? Have you been here long?'

'Two years. I trained at Hampstead,' she said. And she'd loved it there. Until Lucas had crashed his motorbike three and a half years ago, leaving her a widow with a year-old baby. Riding too fast—but not to get home to her. He'd been going too fast because he'd loved the thrill of speed. Because he'd liked taking risks. And either he hadn't seen the icy patch, or he'd thought himself invincible, or maybe both. The end result was the same.

They'd had to airlift him to his own emergency department.

Losing a patient was always tough. But when that patient was a colleague as well, one who was charming and popular with everyone no matter what their qualifications or status… The accident had broken his team as much as it had broken Rebecca. And she hadn't even had a chance to organise the funeral before Fate added another nasty twist. She'd assumed her missed period was because of the stress of the situation; she hadn't even considered she might be pregnant. Being rushed into the same emergency department where Lucas had died and learning that she'd had an ectopic pregnancy—losing one of her fallopian tubes as well as the baby—had been almost too much to bear.

She shook herself. Not now. She'd had three and a half years to get used to being a widow. Three and a half years of learning not to wrap Jasmine completely in cotton wool, not to worry every second they were apart, and not to overcompensate and try to be both parents. Moving to Muswell Hill had really helped her, and Jasmine loved her nursery school. 'Being a male midwife is a fairly unusual career choice,' she said. 'What made you pick midwifery?'

'I used to be a building site manager,' he said.

Site manager to a midwife? That was quite a career change. 'Just as well Mr Brown didn't know you worked on a building site, leaning down from the scaffolding and whistling at every passing woman,' she said. 'He'd have worried even more about letting you near the business end.'

Nathaniel laughed, a rich, deep sound that set those tingles off again. 'That's horrible stereotyping.'

'A bit,' she agreed. 'But whenever I've walked past scaffolding that's what the builders always do.'

'You're blonde and you're pretty. Of course they'll whistle at you.'

She felt her face go pink. 'I wasn't fishing for a compliment. I meant they whistle at *every* passing woman.'

'Not all of them do. Some builders prefer men,' Nathaniel said.

Was that an oblique way of telling her that he was gay? 'OK,' she said carefully. 'So what persuaded you to change careers?'

It was a story Nathaniel was used to telling. 'Fell off a roof,' he said cheerfully. 'Broke my back. I spent four months in hospital.'

'Ouch,' she said. 'And I imagine you must've needed a ton of physio when you left hospital.'

He nodded. 'It gave me a long time to think about what I really wanted to do with my life. Whether I had the nerve to work on a site again, whether I could make myself go up a ladder to check something.'

'Did you?'

'Let's see. Work in an air-conditioned hospital; or be on a site in all weathers, from frost and snow to rain or blazing sun, knowing I'd maybe make it to forty before arthritis started making my job a lot more difficult every day?' He spread his hands. 'It was an easy choice.'

Though not all of the choices had been his. It had been Angela's choice to end their engagement. It had taken him a long time to come to terms with the fact that the love of his life hadn't stuck around when he'd needed her most. Eventually he'd worked out why: she'd agreed to marry Nathaniel the site manager, the man whose career was doing nicely. She hadn't signed up to nurse him through a broken back, not knowing if he'd ever be able to walk again and they'd spend their entire marriage with her as his carer. Even though he understood it, he still found it hard to forgive. And even now he resented the fact that she'd ended their engagement so fast, not even waiting a couple of weeks to see if there were any signs of recovery.

To dump him so swiftly: had she ever really loved him in the first place? Was he that hopeless a judge of character when it came to relationships? The whole situation had really knocked his confidence in himself, and he hadn't had a serious relationship since, not wanting to get close to someone else and risk discovering that he wasn't enough for her, either. He kept his heart under wraps and his relationships short.

Not that he was going to tell Rebecca Hart anything about that. It wasn't relevant to his job. Or to what she'd asked him.

'I wanted a job where I'd make a difference,' he said. 'Where I'd make people's lives better. The nurses on my ward got me through those first rough weeks, and it made me realise how amazing they were. I wanted to be able to do that for someone, too.'

'Nurses are amazing,' she agreed. 'So did you start training as soon as you were back on your feet?'

He nodded. 'I left school at sixteen, so despite having my site manager's qualifications I had to do a year's access course at the university before they'd accept me to do a BSc in nursing.' He smiled. 'I loved the course. I was going to work in the Emergency Department, because that was my favourite placement. But then, in my final year, my best friend's wife was pregnant. Jason was away on business and Denise's family was in Paris, celebrating her aunt's sixtieth birthday—they thought it would be fine to go because all first babies are late and take ages.'

'Right,' Rebecca said, rolling her eyes because she clearly knew how much of a myth that was. 'So I'm guessing she went into labour early?'

'Yes. Her best friend was meant to be her backup birth partner, but she was a junior doctor and was in Theatre when Denise went into labour. Obviously she couldn't just walk out of the op, so Denise called me in a panic. I thought I'd just be there for the first stage of labour and Jason would be back in time for the birth, but it was a quick labour and he didn't make it to the hospital until Sienna was a couple of hours old. It was the most amazing thing in the world, being there when my goddaughter took her first breath.' He grinned. 'The first thing Sienna did after being born was an enormous poo, and my first job as her godfather was to change that nappy.'

Rebecca's blue eyes twinkled. 'Ah, yes, the joys of the first nappy. So even the meconium didn't put you off wanting to be a midwife?'

'Nope. In a weird way, that decided me. Looking at her face, seeing those first few moments, I knew Maternity was where I wanted to be. Which meant I was just about to graduate in the wrong subject.' He wrinkled his nose. 'Well, ish. My degree gave me good foundations for midwifery. After I graduated, I did the eighteen-month short course to become a midwife. I was the only man in my year group, but most people accepted me.'

'Most?'

'One of my tutors didn't really take to me,' he admitted. 'In her view, men shouldn't be midwives because they can't have babies.'

Rebecca winced. 'That's unfair. And also not true—are you going to say heart surgeons can't do their job if they haven't had heart surgery themselves? And what about women who can't have children? That's not a valid reason for them not being midwives.' She looked cross. 'I hate that kind of prejudice.'

And that really gratified him, at the same time as it made him realise that he'd misjudged her. She hadn't stepped in earlier to pull rank; she really had intended to help and be supportive.

He shrugged. 'I guess it helped prepare me for any parents-to-be who thought the same as my tutor did. I learned to come up with some solid answers. But here I am. I qualified, I love my job, and it's such a privilege to help women through one of the most intense and emotional experiences of their lives.'

'Do you get many dads reacting to you the way Mr Brown did today?' she asked.

'One or two. A couple of women have said they didn't want a man delivering their baby— ironically, they ended up with sections and a male surgeon,' he added, rolling his eyes, 'but normally, once people get over the surprise of me not being a woman, they're fine about it. Not many go from nought to shouty in two seconds, the way he did.' He smiled at her. 'What about you? Why did you choose Maternity?'

'It was my favourite rotation,' she said. 'That first moment after the birth, when all's still, and the baby opens their eyes and looks at you, and you see all the wonder of the universe in their face.'

'Those tiny fingers and tiny toes,' he said. 'I *love* babies' feet. And the way babies grip your finger.'

'The softness of their skin,' Rebecca said. 'Even if they're a late baby and a bit over-cooked, or an early baby covered in vernix—they're just *beautiful*.'

And that look of joy on her face took his breath away, transforming her from the slightly starchy doctor he'd first met to the most gorgeous woman he'd even seen. His spine pricked with awareness of her.

'I think,' Nathan said, 'we're on the same page.'

'I agree.' She smiled. 'Thank you for the coffee, Mr Jones.'

'Nathaniel.' He waited a beat. Was she going to stay all starchy and formal? Or would she…?

'Rebecca.'

Only then did he realise he'd been holding his breath. Which was crazy.

'I'm afraid I need to get going—but welcome to the team.'

'Cheers,' he said, and deliberately stayed to finished his own coffee.

He was so aware of the brilliant sky blue of her eyes, and the way her hair—even caught back in a ponytail for work—looked like sunlight on ripened cornfields. The shape of her mouth.

Although he'd dated a few times since the end of his engagement, there hadn't been anyone serious and it had been a long while since he'd felt that instant zing of attraction. He'd just been going through the motions, doing what everyone expected of him.

He hadn't been able to help himself glancing at Rebecca's left hand as they chatted. No ring, though that meant nothing nowadays. For all he knew, she could be in a committed relationship but hadn't formalised it. Though he wasn't going to ask any of his colleagues if she was single; the last thing he wanted was to put either of them under the focus of the hospital rumour mill.

She hadn't flirted with him; but he hadn't been able to stop himself flirting a bit with her.

He was really going to have to be careful.

CHAPTER TWO

NATHANIEL MANAGED TO keep himself in check the next day, more by luck than judgement because his path didn't actually cross Rebecca's. But on Thursday he had a patient who worried him. It should've been a routine thirty-four-week antenatal appointment, but Josette Kamanya's blood pressure was a bit high for his liking. And his worries increased when he tested her urine sample and the dipstick showed the presence of protein. Her BMI was more than thirty-five, she'd had high blood pressure before getting pregnant, and this was her first baby; an alarm bell began to ring in the back of his head. Particularly when she admitted to having had a few headaches recently. 'But that's all just a part of pregnancy, isn't it?' she asked.

Yes, but the symptoms were adding up to something he really wasn't happy about.

'Mrs Kamanya, would you mind if I had a look at your feet?' he asked.

She looked surprised but nodded and slipped her feet out of her shoes.

'Your ankles and feet look a little bit swollen to me,' he said. That was another sign that worried him.

'It's probably just because I've been walking about a lot and it's been hot for June,' she said.

He wasn't convinced. 'What about your hands and fingers?' he asked gently. 'Have your rings started to feel tight or anything like that?'

'I guess they have, in the last couple of days,' she admitted.

The alarm bells in his head grew a bit louder.

'Have you felt any pain in your tummy or under your ribs?'

'No.'

He smiled. 'That's good. Have you had any feelings of nausea, or actually been sick?'

'No, thankfully,' she said, looking relieved. 'That was all over weeks ago.'

'Glad to hear it. Going back to those headaches you mentioned—have you noticed any flashing lights, or any blurriness in your vision?'

'No. I don't get migraines or anything like that,' she said. 'It's just a headache that's been a bit hard to shift.'

Nathaniel still wasn't happy. Often women with pre-eclampsia felt perfectly fine and it was only the urine test and blood pressure result that indicated there was a problem.

'Has anyone in your family ever had pre-eclampsia?' he asked.

'I don't think my mum had any problems when she had me. I'm an only child, but I can't remember any of my cousins having a problem, either.' She looked at him, biting her lip. 'Is something wrong?'

'I think,' he said, 'you might have a condition called pre-eclampsia, but I want to talk to one of the doctors. Would you mind if I brought someone else in to see you?'

Her eyes widened. 'Is there something wrong with my baby?'

He held her hand. No medic could ever promise that everything was going to be a hundred per cent fine, but he didn't want her worrying. 'It's not that. If I'm right in my suspicions and you have pre-eclampsia, it's a very common condition, and we're used to treating it. You're in absolutely the right place and we're going to look after you both,' he said.

'All right,' she said, but she still looked anxious.

'I'll be back really quickly. Have a sip or two of water, and I'd like you to try some breathing exercises for me while you're waiting.' Those at least he knew would help. 'Rest your hands at the bottom of your ribcage so your fingertips are just touching,' he said, and she followed his directions. 'That's perfect, Mrs Kamanya.' He smiled at her. 'Breathe in for a slow count of five, and your fingertips should move apart. Now breathe out for a slow count of five, and your fingertips should come back together again. That's brilliant.' He smiled again. 'I'd like you to do fifty breaths in and out like that, and I'll be back before you know it. Is that OK?'

'All right,' she said, clearly worrying but trying to be brave.

The only one in the doctors' office was Rebecca. Given their talk the other day, he hoped she'd be supportive rather than trying to take over or dismissing his fears; though it didn't help that the little flare of attraction grew brighter when he saw her. 'Reb—' He stopped himself. They'd been on first-name terms the other day in the canteen, but she might prefer formality on the ward itself. 'Dr Hart, can I ask you to come and see one of my mums, please?'

'Rebecca,' she said. 'I prefer working on first-name terms.'

'Nathaniel,' he said.

'What's wrong, Nathaniel?'

Weird how hearing her use his given name for the first time made a little prickle go all the way up his spine. He shook himself. He was here for his mum-to-be, not himself. 'I think Josette Kamanya might have pre-eclampsia.' He gave Rebecca a quick rundown of the case. 'She's had high blood pressure since before she was pregnant, and according to her notes this is the first appointment where she's had protein in her urine. But I've just got a funny feeling about it.'

'You're probably right. I always trust a midwife's instinct,' Rebecca said.

Good. So this wasn't going to be another power struggle. He'd been right in his revised assessment of her. 'Thank you.' He walked with her to the antenatal clinic room. 'How are you doing, Mrs Kamanya?'

'I just did breath number fifty,' she said.

'Perfect timing, then.' He introduced Rebecca swiftly.

'Mr Jones is a little bit concerned about how you're doing, so he asked me to come and see you, Mrs Kamanya,' Rebecca said.

'So what exactly is this pre-eclampsia thing, Dr Hart?' Mrs Kamanya asked.

'It's a condition that affects mums and babies and often starts after the twenty-week mark. It's quite common—about one in twenty mums has it—so don't get too alarmed,' she reassured Mrs Kamanya. 'Usually our first clue is when you have high blood pressure and protein in your urine. We think it's to do with the blood vessels in the placenta not developing properly, so the placenta doesn't send as much blood as it should do to the baby.'

'Is the baby going to be all right?' Mrs Kamanya asked.

'You and the baby should both be just fine, but if we don't keep a close eye on you and treat you then there is a risk of you developing complications,' Rebecca said.

'What sort of complications?' Mrs Kamanya asked.

'There can be a problem with your blood clotting, or you could go on to develop a condition called eclampsia, where you might start having fits. You're also at a higher risk of having a stroke,' Nathaniel explained. 'Which I know sounds scary, but if we start treating you now all the risks go way down.'

'So I agree with Mr Jones that we need to keep an eye on you and the baby,' Rebecca said. 'I'd like to do some blood tests to check your liver and kidney function and make sure your blood's clotting properly. I'd also like him to monitor the baby's heartbeat—which won't hurt either of you; we'll give you an ultrasound so we can take a closer look at how the placenta's doing; and we'll give you a blood test to check levels of a hormone called placental growth factor, which will help me diagnose whether this is pre-eclampsia or not. Is that OK with you?'

Mrs Kamanya nodded.

Rebecca checked the notes Nathaniel had made. 'Your blood pressure's a bit on the high side for my liking, so I'd also like to give you some medication to lower it. It's safe for pregnant women to take, but you might have some side effects.' Between them, she and Nathaniel ran through the side effects.

Mrs Kamanya bit her lip. 'I really don't like the idea of taking medication while I'm pregnant. And I'm worried that it might hurt the baby.'

'It's your choice,' Rebecca said gently, 'but without the medication there's a risk that your blood pressure could go up further, and that's more likely to cause complications which will be more of a risk to the baby.'

'So there isn't really a choice.'

Rebecca took her hand and squeezed it. 'You can change your mind at any time, Mrs Kamanya. It's fine. This is all about making you comfortable and keeping you well. Plus we'll be here with you, so if you decide to have the medication and you start to feel any side effects, you can tell us and we can do something to help—including giving you a different medication.'

'You'll be here with me?' Mrs Kamanya's eyes widened as she took in what Rebecca had said. 'Do you mean I'll have to stay in hospital?'

'For a couple of days, yes,' Rebecca said. 'We'll see how things go. It might be that we send you home in a couple of days under strict instructions to rest, and to call us straight away if you're worried about anything. But, like Mr Jones, I'd be happier if you were admitted for the next couple of days so we can keep a close eye on you and the baby.' She paused. 'There is one thing. If you do have pre-eclampsia, and we can't get your blood pressure to settle, we might need to deliver the baby a bit earlier than planned.'

'But I'm only thirty-four weeks pregnant!' Mrs Kamanya looked shocked. 'That's way too soon.'

'We'll see what the tests say,' Rebecca said, 'but if we do have to deliver the baby early, we'll make sure you have steroids to help mature the baby's lungs and minimise any risks to both of you. The main thing is that we look after you both properly.'

'I've had my labour bag packed for weeks—

everyone at my antenatal group has—but I never dreamed...' Mrs Kamanya shook her head. 'I can't have the baby yet. I just *can't*.'

'Try not to worry,' Nathaniel said. 'I know that's easier said than done, but you're in the right place.'

'So why did I get pre-eclampsia? Is it something I did wrong?' Mrs Kamanya asked.

'It's nothing you've done. We don't know the exact causes,' Rebecca said. 'The risk factors include having high blood pressure and a family history of pre-eclampsia—not just your family, but including if your partner's mother had pre-eclampsia—or if you have an auto-immune disease such as lupus or antiphospholipid syndrome.'

'I don't have a family history and neither does Andras, as far as I know. And I don't have any other diseases. I've felt perfectly fit and well.' She bit her lip. 'Will the baby be OK?'

'The baby's going to be just fine, because we'll be monitoring you both,' Nathan reassured her.

'Will I get this pre-eclampsia again, if I have another baby?' Mrs Kamanya asked.

'You're at a greater risk of having high blood pressure and developing pre-eclampsia in your next pregnancy, yes. But it doesn't mean that you'll definitely get them, just that the risk will be a bit higher and we'll keep a closer eye on you,' Rebecca said, squeezing her hand. 'We're going to look after you, and it's your job to get plenty of rest.'

'I'm not very good at resting,' Mrs Kamanya said ruefully.

'Me, neither. I was a total nightmare during my pregnancy. And the worst thing was when people nagged me to put my feet up and *rest.*' Rebecca rolled her eyes and grimaced. 'It drove me crazy and I used to remind them that "rest" is technically a four-letter word.'

During her pregnancy?

Rebecca had a child?

Again, Nathaniel found himself glancing at her left hand to double-check. Definitely no ring. Was she still in a relationship with the father of her baby, or was she a single parent?

There was absolutely no way he could ask without being rude. He'd have to think of a tactful way to broach the subject.

'But, much as I sympathise with you and I'd hate it if I were in your shoes, I'm afraid I'm going to have to tell you to rest,' Rebecca continued, smiling at Mrs Kamanya. 'Is there anyone we can call for you to go and fetch your things?'

'Andras—my husband—is in meetings all day.' Mrs Kamanya shook her head. 'If I call my mum she'd never stop fussing over me and it'd drive me mad, being wrapped in cotton wool. My best friend's a teacher so she can't just ask for time off whenever she feels like it.' She grimaced. 'And my mother-in-law would start wringing her hands and making it all about her.'

'That kind of drama makes it hard for anyone to rest,' Rebecca agreed.

Nathaniel wondered if she was talking from personal experience, or from what she'd observed on the ward.

'Perhaps we can call your husband or your best friend during their lunch break, and they can bring some things in for you this evening,' Nathaniel suggested.

'That would be good. Thank you.' Mrs Kamanya bit her lip. 'If I do have to have the baby early…that doesn't mean I have to have a section, does it?'

'We might be able to induce you,' Rebecca said, 'but I think it's a good idea to prepare yourself for the possibility of having a section. But it's really not as bad as you think. Women recover much quicker nowadays than they did twenty years ago. You're not going to be stuck at home for months, unable to drive and having to rely on everyone else to lift things for you.'

Mrs Kamanya didn't look convinced.

'Maybe we can get one of the mums here who's had a section to come and have a chat with you and tell you what it's really like,' Nathaniel said. 'That way, you won't be guessing and worrying and making it scarier than it really is.'

'I suppose,' Mrs Kamanya said.

'Nathaniel will get you booked onto the ward, and I'll get everything written up so we can run the tests,' Rebecca said.

'And we're here to answer any questions,' Nathaniel said. 'Not just us—all the midwives and doctors on the ward. We'd all much rather you asked us whatever you want to know than just kept worrying in silence.'

Rebecca smiled at her. 'As Mr Jones said, try not to worry. You're in good hands with him.'

She was completely different from how she'd been the other day. And Nathaniel liked the fact that she put their mums first. He liked *her*.

But he couldn't get involved with her. Even if she didn't have a partner, she had a child; she had commitments. The little voice in his head added a sharp reminder: he hadn't been enough for Angie, back in the days when he was getting on in his career, so what made him think that a junior midwife could be enough for a successful senior doctor? He needed to put a lid on his attraction to her.

He sorted out the blood samples Rebecca had asked for, organised an MRI and set up the cardiotocography to measure the baby's heartbeat and keep a trace for the file. Then he took Mrs Kamanya through to the ward and got her settled in, organised the monitoring he wanted done for the rest of the day, and asked Gurleen, who was on the reception desk, to get in touch with Mrs Kamanya's husband and best friend.

When his clinic was over, he dropped in to the ward to see how Mrs Kamanya was doing. Rebecca was there, sitting next to the bed, talking to her and making her laugh.

He blinked in surprise. 'I didn't expect to see you here.'

'It's my lunch break,' Rebecca explained. 'And I remember what it was like to be told to rest and being desperate for someone to take my mind off things.'

'Distraction is good.' Though he hadn't expected this sort of kindness from her. Then he made the mistake of meeting her eye, and the attraction he'd been trying to suppress turned into a hot, heady pulse. Oh, for pity's sake. Now wasn't the time or the place.

'Dr Hart's been so kind,' Mrs Kamanya said.

He opened his mouth, intending to say something anodyne, but what came out was, 'Don't tell her this, but she's my favourite out of the doctors on the ward.'

Oh, no. Earth, open and swallow me now, he begged silently.

Rebecca shocked him even more. 'Don't tell him this,' she said in a stage whisper, 'but he's as good as a woman when it comes to being a midwife.'

And she gave him the cheekiest, cheekiest grin—one which turned that flicker of attraction into a raging fire in an instant.

If someone had picked them both up right now and dropped them on a deserted island, he would've kissed her until they were both dizzy.

But this was work, and they needed to concentrate on their mum-to-be. 'Is there anything I can get you, Mrs Kamanya?' he asked.

She shook her head. 'Thanks, but I'm fine. That nice woman on reception talked to my husband and my best friend. Andras is going to move one of his meetings so he can go home and fetch my labour bag, and my best friend's coming in straight after school finishes so she can take over—well, babysitting me, I guess.' She rolled her eyes.

'That's good,' Nathaniel said.

'And, meanwhile, we're talking sudoku,' Rebecca said with a smile. 'Want to join us?'

He held up his hands in a surrender gesture.

'Number puzzles are not my thing at all. If it was a pool table, you're on. Or a quiz team where someone else gets to do the literature questions and I can do sports, TV and music. But those?' He nodded at the magazine. 'Count me out.'

'Nice pun, Mr Jones,' Mrs Kamanya said, laughing.

'Quiz team,' Rebecca said thoughtfully. 'We can always use someone good for the ward quiz team. We have a monthly quiz in the pub with Paediatrics and the Emergency Department— and we're a bit overdue a win.'

'Are you asking me to join the team?'

Oh, for crying out loud. Why had he opened his mouth? He'd practically purred it at her, as if he were teasing her about asking him on a date. This was nothing of the sort. It was a team thing.

But she didn't look awkward or embarrassed. She just smiled. 'Yes. But you'd better be good, or you'll be buying everyone cake to make up for it.'

'That,' Mrs Kamanya said, 'sounds like an excellent idea.' She gave Rebecca a high-five.

This was a side of Rebecca he hadn't seen. Playful, fun. And he really, *really* liked it.

'Let me know when the next quiz is and I'm in—as long as I'm not on duty,' he said.

'Sure,' she said.

That smile made his heart feel as if it had done a backflip. An anatomically impossible backflip, but a backflip all the same. 'I'll see you both later,' he said.

At the end of his shift, Nathaniel checked in with Mrs Kamanya again; her best friend was with her and she seemed a lot more settled. And then he headed for Rebecca's office. She was clearly finishing off some paperwork.

'Hi,' he said.

She looked up from her computer. 'Hi.'

'I just wanted to say thanks for all your help with Mrs Kamanya today,' he said.

'That's what I'm here for. To support my team when things get complicated.'

Yeah. He'd definitely misinterpreted the way she'd come in to bat his corner with Mike Brown.

Her smile was warm and inviting, and even though he'd had every intention of keeping his distance he just couldn't resist asking, 'Do you fancy grabbing a pizza with me after work to-night?'

'I… Thank you for asking, but I have commitments,' she said, clearly choosing her words carefully.

'Your partner would be welcome to join

us, of course.' Oh, way to go, Nathaniel. Subtle. *Not*.

'No partner,' she said.

And that changed everything. If she didn't have a partner, there was no barrier to them getting to know each other better. 'Then maybe we could have that pizza another evening?'

She took a deep breath. 'It's kind of you to ask me—' Kindness hadn't even been in the running order of reasons why he'd asked. '—but I don't date.'

So it wasn't personal? Not like Angie. And that gave him the courage to say, 'May I ask why?'

'I'm a widow,' she said, 'and I don't want to get involved with anyone.'

Rebecca was very young to be a widow. Though Nathaniel wasn't going to be crass enough to ask what had happened. Plus it was none of his business. But he still wondered why she didn't date. Was she still grieving for her husband? Did she think nobody would match up to his memory? Or had her marriage been unhappy and she didn't want to get involved in another potentially difficult relationship? Not that he could ask. That was way, way too intrusive.

'I'm sorry,' she said. 'I have a daughter who's almost five, and she comes first.'

'Of course.'

'I'm not looking to date anyone,' she said. 'But friendship—that's a different thing. I'm happy to be friends.'

'Friends,' he said, deliberately keeping his voice neutral and non-judgemental.

'I'm sorry I can't offer you anything else.'

So was he. But he wasn't going to blank her just because she'd turned him down. 'Friendship is fine by me,' he said. And, wanting to make her feel more comfortable, he added, 'Maybe we can do the pizza as a team thing.'

She smiled. 'That'd be good.'

'OK. See you later,' he said, and left before he could make even more of an idiot of himself than he already had.

Rebecca stared out of the door after Nathaniel.

It was the first time anyone had asked her out since Lucas.

Six and a half years.

In some ways, it was flattering; in others, it was terrifying. No way could she risk dating again. She had Jasmine to think of; and her daughter would come first. Always. And, apart from that, she'd learned her lesson well. She'd married someone gorgeous and charming, someone who'd swept her off her feet and they'd got married six months after they'd first met. Not long after their first anniversary, she realised she'd made a mistake; Lucas was an adrenalin junkie who didn't get enough thrills even from his high-pressure job, and he'd put his need for adventure before everything else. The thrill of the chase had worn off very quickly for him, to the point where he seemed to prefer the company of his friends to hers, and she'd been seriously considering leaving him when she'd found out that she was pregnant.

The news had meant she'd stayed, wanting to give their baby a chance to be part of a family. Lucas had promised to change. She knew he'd tried—but he'd been so bored by domestic life. He'd hated the day-to-day grind of life with a small baby, with the nappy-changing and the crying and the lack of sleep. Even when Rebecca had sent him off climbing at the weekends with his like-minded friends, it hadn't been enough; he'd felt guilty about leaving her to cope with the baby on her own. And that guilt had come further and further between them, leading him to do more and more reckless things.

Including buying the expensive motorbike that had ultimately claimed his life.

Rebecca sat back in her chair, no longer seeing the words on her computer screen.

She hadn't been enough to soothe Lucas's

restlessness, and nor had fatherhood. Even if he'd survived the crash, even if he'd been able to go back to work afterwards and back to riding his motorbike, she was pretty sure that she and Jasmine wouldn't have been enough for Lucas. He'd needed more than their little family unit: he'd craved the adrenalin rush of danger. She'd suspected that Lucas had also found female distractions elsewhere since she'd fallen pregnant—though she'd never asked, never accused, because she hadn't wanted to rock the boat. Not when she was heavily pregnant, or sleep-deprived with a newborn, and too tired for a fight. Though she had been starting to think that maybe she and Jasmine would be better off on their own. That Lucas needed his freedom much more than he needed a family.

She'd actually planned to sit down with him that night and suggest it. She'd fallen asleep on the sofa, waiting for him to come home.

And then the police had called round to see her and everything had changed…

She didn't want to risk her heart again. To risk falling for another Mr Wrong, especially when she had her daughter to consider. Yes, Nathan seemed a nice guy; but charming men could always seem to be whatever you wanted them to be. Who was to say he wouldn't change, the way Lucas had, once she'd given him what he wanted?

Plus, if he wanted children of his own, what then? She'd lost one of her fallopian tubes as a result of the ectopic pregnancy. Even getting pregnant again might be an issue, and if she did conceive then her risk of having another ectopic pregnancy was greater than average. Was it fair to get involved with someone who might want kids of his own when she might not be able to give him a family?

So it was better to stay single. To keep her heart intact. To focus on the important things in her life: her daughter, her family and her job.

Saying no had been the right thing to do.

And those wistful 'what ifs' trying to fight through her heart were just going to have to stay buried.

CHAPTER THREE

NATHANIEL WAS OFF duty on Friday, which gave him plenty of time to brood. Going for a run didn't help; he couldn't settle to watching a movie, so in the end he cleaned his flat, deciding that his least favourite chore suited his mood. Why had he been so stupid, giving in to that mad impulse to ask Rebecca out? Why hadn't he waited, let them get to know each other a bit better first? Even though he'd covered over the immediate awkwardness by suggesting that they did the pizza as a team thing, he knew he'd rushed it.

Would she give him a second chance, maybe a bit later? Or had he ruined it for himself by asking too soon?

And why was he asking her, in any case?

'I need my head examining,' he told Leo, his Bengal cat.

Leo patted Nathaniel's hand with his paw.

Nathaniel smiled. There was probably more

sense in his hand right now than there was in his head. Rebecca had already told him she didn't date. Even if she changed her mind, he didn't do serious relationships. Angie had dumped him while he'd still been up to his eyeballs in painkillers. He didn't want to get involved with someone, lose his heart to her and then discover he wasn't enough for *her* to love, either.

Yet he couldn't stop thinking about Rebecca. He didn't really understand why. He hadn't even liked her when he'd first met her. He'd thought she was the sort who pulled rank and interfered. But how she'd been with one of their higher-risk mums, listening and even spending her lunch break with Mrs Kamanya to cheer her up, had shown him that Rebecca Hart had a kind, soft heart.

Plus she was gorgeous. All that straight blonde hair she kept tied back for work, and eyes the colour of a summer sky.

Why was it getting to him just now? It wasn't an anniversary or anything like that. And he knew what his big sister would say when he turned up with flowers and a punnet of those candyfloss grapes she'd been scoffing for England since getting pregnant. He could even hear Charlotte's voice echoing in his head: 'Nate, you're thirty-four years old. Young, gorgeous and single. The world should be your oyster.'

The life he had now wasn't what he'd planned at all. Nine years ago, he'd been looking forward to a summer wedding with everyone dancing at the reception in a rose garden; he was doing well at work; and he'd been thinking about the two kids he and Angie were going to have—a boy first, then a girl.

And then he'd fallen off a roof.

One little slip and his whole word had shattered.

No wedding and no babies.

The nearest he was going to get were his goddaughter, his niece-to-be, and the babies he delivered on the ward.

He told himself he was fine with that. He *liked* the new life he'd made for himself. He had a close family, great friends, and a really rewarding job.

'So why, this week, doesn't it feel enough?' he asked the cat, who just stared at him with huge green eyes.

He wasn't still in love with Angie. He'd been hurt and angry and desolate for a while, but he'd finally come round to thinking that she'd done them both a favour. If she couldn't stick around when the going got tough, at least they didn't have two kids whose lives would be ripped apart in a break-up.

But it had also left him unable to trust. Unable to trust himself—how had he managed to pick someone so wrong for him?—and unable to trust that whoever he dated might really love him. Or had the problem been him, all along? If he hadn't been enough for Angie, how could he be enough for anyone else?

Enough brooding, he told himself. He needed to go and buy flowers. And he'd try to get Rebecca's smile out of his head. He really needed to stop wanting things he couldn't have.

Rebecca curled up on the sofa with a mug of tea. She really wasn't following the plot of the film she'd been trying to watch. Mainly because she couldn't get Nathaniel Jones out of her head.

Should she have said yes when he'd asked her out? She knew what her best friends and family would say. At the age of thirty-four, she was still young enough to have fun, and she shouldn't spend the rest of her life in mourning for Lucas.

She could almost hear her little sister's voice. 'You need something for you, too. You're more than just Jasmine's mum or my sister or Dr Hart. You're Rebecca, too. And it'd be good for you to have a night off. This guy didn't ask you to marry him, he asked you to go out on a *date*. There's a difference.'

But there was a good reason why she'd said no. Lots of good reasons. The first of which was that she'd made a huge mistake with Lucas. She'd loved him, but she shouldn't have married him in a rush like that, and she didn't want to make the same kind of mistake in any future relationships. She didn't want to end up with someone else who didn't think she was enough. It wouldn't be fair to Jasmine, either.

And even if she did find someone who loved her for herself, who wanted to make a future with her and be a stepdad to Jasmine, there were other hurdles. Supposing he wanted children and she couldn't have them?

No. She'd made the right decision in turning him down.

Though she couldn't help wondering, what if? What if she'd said yes? What if she'd let herself have a nice evening, got to know him better and then decided if she wanted to repeat it?

Dating.

Opening herself up to a relationship again.

It was a terrifying proposition.

It could be so easy.

But she would be opening herself up to a world where she could get hurt again. A world where she'd be found wanting. A world where she'd fail.

It was too much of a risk.

Yes, Nathaniel Jones was cute; his dark eyes had the longest lashes she'd ever seen on a man. His mouth was beautiful. Then she wished she hadn't thought about his mouth, because her thoughts immediately rushed on to the next stage—wondering what his mouth might feel like against hers.

For pity's sake. She was thirty-four, not fourteen. Mooning over a good-looking man wasn't the sort of thing she should be doing.

But all the same she found herself thinking about Nathaniel later that night, going over and over the same questions. Had she been too hasty in turning him down? Should she have agreed to go out with him? Could she take the risk of dating again?

On Monday morning, Nathaniel was in the middle of writing up notes when Rebecca came to find him. 'I know you're rostered on the labour ward, this morning, Nathaniel, but I was wondering how many ECVs you'd done?'

An ECV or external cephalic version was a procedure used to turn a breech baby in the womb. 'I've seen a couple, but not actually done any myself,' he said. 'Is that what you're doing today?'

She nodded. 'If you'd like to assist—or even do the ECV yourself, if my mum's happy for that to happen—you'd be very welcome.'

'I'd love to.' And it warmed him that she'd thought of him.

'Great. I'll come and find you at half-past ten, and maybe you can do the initial checks for me and talk my mum through the procedure.'

'You're on.'

She was as good as her word and came to find him at half-past ten. 'So you're clear on how the procedure works?'

'Yes.'

'Great. You take the lead, and I'll be there as backup. I've already checked with the Ridleys and they're both quite happy for you to do the procedure.'

Nathaniel had already arranged for a colleague to look after his mums-to-be while he was working with Rebecca, so he followed her to the consultation room.

She introduced him to the couple sitting on the bed. 'Mr and Mrs Ridley, this is Nathaniel Jones, who'll be doing the procedure this morning.'

'Nice to meet you, Mr Jones,' Mrs Ridley replied, smiling.

'Nathaniel, this is Mr and Mrs Ridley. Mrs Ridley's thirty-six weeks right now and the baby's decided to stay feet-first.' Rebecca smiled and gestured to him to take over.

'Lovely to meet you both,' Nathaniel said. 'It's really common for a baby to be feet-first or bottom-first in your pelvis during pregnancy, but most of them have turned head-down by this point. I'm assuming you've both already talked this through with Dr Hart and you've decided to have an ECV in the hope the baby will do a somersault in the womb, so he or she will be born head-first rather than feet-first and you're more likely to have a normal birth?'

Mrs Ridley nodded. 'Dr Hart's warned us there's a fifty-fifty chance of it working, and if it doesn't work then I'd like to try for a vaginal breech birth. I'd rather not have a section, though I realise that might have to happen if we can't make a normal birth work.'

'Some babies are stubborn and turn all the way back again a few days after they've turned head-first,' Nathaniel said. 'And there's also a small chance that we might have to deliver the baby today, if we're not happy with the baby's heartbeat afterwards or if there's any bleeding from your placenta.'

'We're prepared for that,' Mr Ridley said, indicating a labour bag.

'Great. And I'm also assuming that you don't have pre-eclampsia, you're not having twins, the baby isn't small for dates, you haven't had any recent bleeding and your waters haven't broken,' Nathaniel said, mentally ticking off all the criteria.

Rebecca's approving smile meant he'd remembered all the contraindications for the procedure.

When Mrs Ridley nodded, he said, 'So what happens now is we'll do a scan to confirm the baby's position and the position of your placenta, as well as the amount of amniotic fluid.' He smiled. 'Then I'll check your blood pressure and your pulse, and check the baby's heart rate. Once we're happy everything's as it should be, Dr Hart will give you a small injection to help relax the muscles in your uterus. The medication won't affect the baby, and there's no risk to you or the baby, but it might make you feel a bit shaky and you might be aware of your heart beating a bit faster.'

'The medication wears off in three minutes,' Rebecca added, 'but it increases the chance of us turning the baby successfully.'

'Can I just double-check your blood group?' Nathaniel asked.

'A positive,' Mrs Ridley said.

'Excellent.' As her blood type wasn't rhesus negative, he knew that meant they wouldn't need to give her an injection of anti-D to stop antibodies forming against the baby's potential rhesus positive blood cells.

The scan confirmed that the baby was breech, and Nathaniel was happy with the position of the placenta and the amniotic fluid level. He checked Mrs Ridley's blood pressure and pulse. 'Perfect,' he said. And the baby's heartbeat was absolutely fine, too.

'Between us, we're going to persuade the baby to do a forward roll,' Rebecca said. 'The whole thing should take about ten minutes, and it might be a little bit uncomfortable. But it shouldn't be painful, so if it hurts you need to tell us immediately and we'll stop.'

'Got it,' Mrs Ridley said.

Rebecca prepared the syringe. 'You'll feel a sharp scratch,' she said, and administered the injection. 'Try to relax your tummy muscles for us, Mrs Ridley.' She turned to Nathaniel. 'So now you put your hands on Mrs Ridley's abdomen, under the baby's bottom, and gently manipulate until you feel the baby starting to move forward. Mrs Ridley, are you comfortable?' she checked.

'I am,' Mrs Ridley confirmed.

'Mr Ridley, you're doing OK?'

Nathaniel liked the fact that Rebecca was

considering the feelings of everyone in the room. Her calmness and capability meant that everyone was relaxed, even though this wasn't a hugely common procedure.

Rebecca directed his movements quietly, and then he felt the baby shift under his hands and do a forward roll.

'Oh!' Mrs Ridley said, sounding surprised. 'I felt the baby turn!'

'And you should feel quite a bit more comfortable, now the baby's head is no longer under your ribcage,' Rebecca said with a smile.

'Oh, I do,' Mrs Ridley said feelingly, rubbing a hand along her ribcage.

'We're going to do another scan now,' Nathaniel said. 'And then we're going to monitor the baby's heart rate for about thirty minutes, to check the baby's comfortable.'

'That's amazing. And it's so much easier not having the baby's head pushing under my ribs,' Mrs Ridley said.

The scan and the monitoring were both satisfactory, to Nathaniel's relief.

'It's all good,' Nathaniel said. 'You're free to go home now, and we'll see you back here in a week. But if you get any vaginal bleeding, or your waters break, or you get painful contractions, or the baby doesn't move as much as normal, then I want you to call us straight away.'

'We will,' Mr Ridley confirmed.

Once the Ridleys had left, Nathaniel turned to Rebecca. 'Thank you. That was amazing.'

'You're welcome. You did a great job—you were calm, you explained everything well, and you did the movements perfectly.'

'I appreciate you giving me the chance to do the ECV myself.'

'Pleasure.' She smiled at him. 'I guess I'd better let you get back to the ward.'

'I guess. Catch you later,' he said.

Rebecca watched Nathaniel leave the room. He'd been really good, calm and reassuring. All the way through the half-hour monitoring after the ECV, he'd chatted to the Ridleys to make sure they were both relaxed and comfortable. He was patient and kind with their parents-to-be, and in a weird way that made Rebecca feel safe with him. As if she could rely on him and he wouldn't let her down, the way Lucas often had.

Not all men were like Lucas.

So maybe she could take a risk.

Maybe she could ask him out for a drink.

Tomorrow, she promised herself, and got on with writing up her notes.

CHAPTER FOUR

REBECCA DIDN'T ACTUALLY see Nathaniel on Tuesday or Wednesday, because their shifts clashed, and on Thursday morning she came in to overhear Amara, one of the younger midwives, who was married to their newest junior doctor, saying to Nathaniel, 'Tanvir's gone down with that gastro bug. There's no way he's going to be able to do the abseil on Saturday.'

She knew Tanvir had organised a team of ten to abseil down one of the buildings in Central London, to raise money for a new scanner for the ward.

'If we don't have the full team, the organisers might not let us do the abseil,' Nathaniel said. 'Maybe I can persuade them to let one of us do it twice. Or…' He looked at Rebecca. 'Dr Hart.' He gave her the sweetest smile. 'How are you with heights?'

She stared at him. 'You're asking *me* to step into Tan's place?'

'It's only a few minutes out of your day. You'll have the most amazing views over the city.'

'And that building is a hundred times my height.' She shook her head. 'Tan asked me a month ago when he first organised it. I said no then, and I'm saying no now.' She couldn't quite believe this. 'I had no idea Tan had talked you into it.'

'My very first day on the team,' he said with a smile. 'And he talked me into being his second in command, so as he's sick it's up to me to fix this.'

'But you hurt yourself falling off a roof. How can you *possibly* offer to walk off the edge of a roof and go down the side of a really tall building, after *that*?' The idea was horrifying.

'My back's all fixed, now.' He shrugged. 'And mentally I'm doing OK. It'll be good for me. I know there will be ropes and a lot of safety requirements, so there's nothing to worry about.'

It sounded to her as if she'd just met another Lucas. Her late husband would've loved the thrill of walking backwards over the edge and then abseiling as fast as he could down one of the biggest structures in London; the sponsorship money and what it would do for the ward would've been incidental to him.

Surely Nathaniel could see the risks, the way she did? Or had she been the one out of step, rather than Lucas?

'Sorry. I can't do it. I've never abseiled before,' she said.

'It's easy. Just don't look down, and think about the money it'll raise for the ward.'

'You're asking me to abseil down one of the tallest buildings in London,' she reminded him.

'With safety ropes,' he pointed out. 'I'm not suggesting you walk a high wire between buildings without a safety rope—or even a little rope off the ground, without a net.'

At least he was acknowledging the need for safety. But it wasn't enough. She shook her head. 'It's still a risk. I'm a single mum. I can't take that kind of risk.'

'When Tan first asked me, I said no,' Nathaniel said. 'All I could see were the risks. I remember what it feels like to fall off a roof. I remember what it feels like to land. And I've pretty much avoided heights ever since. But then I thought about it. This is a really good way to overcome those lingering fears. I'll have to walk over the edge—but I'll be in a safe environment. So it helps me and it helps the ward. Double win.'

Oh. So he *did* see how terrifying it was. And he was trying to face his fears. Move on.

Was it time she did the same?

Take a risk.

'Can I think about it?' she asked.

'Sure,' he said. 'I'm going to call them during my break this morning to see what our options are.' He paused. 'Tell you what. Have lunch with me, and we'll talk about it then.'

'Aren't you on the labour ward this morning?'

'Nope. That's Amara. I'm on clinic,' he said. 'So. Lunch. And you can talk babies to me.'

Was he flirting with her? The way he'd said it, it was as if the words meant something completely different. The base of her neck felt hot. 'I'll come and find you,' she mumbled. 'Better get to my own clinic.'

She managed to put Nathaniel out of her mind during clinic, but then it was lunchtime. When she went to find him, he'd just finished writing up notes.

'Lunch is on me,' he said. 'Not because I'm trying to make you feel beholden to me, or to guilt you into agreeing to do it.'

No, but she suspected he intended to charm her into it. And she'd learned the hard way that charm wasn't enough. It faded and left resentment in its place. 'I'd rather go halves,' she said.

'Is it that scary, someone buying you a coffee and a sandwich?' he asked.

Yes. 'No,' she fibbed.

'Well, then. Let me buy you a sandwich, and we'll talk babies.' He smiled. 'There aren't any strings.'

'Just abseiling ropes.'

'Yes, but the sandwich isn't dependent on that. It's just lunch, Dr Hart.'

She knew he'd deliberately used her title rather than her first name, to remind her of their formal working relationship. Making a fuss would be ridiculous. Plus part of her really did want to have lunch with him, get to know him a bit better. She gave in. 'All right. Thank you.'

In the canteen, she chose a tuna salad sandwich on seeded wholemeal bread, and a skinny cappuccino. He kept the conversation to work, but she knew she owed him an answer about Saturday. 'What did the abseil people say?' she asked.

'We can still go ahead, but I need to give them the name of a replacement team member.'

And if she took too long giving him an answer, that wouldn't give him enough time to find a replacement for Tan. It was too short notice.

'Why are you doing the abseil?' she asked.

He shrugged. 'To raise money for the scanner. To feel part of the team.'

Which was fair enough, but worry still nagged at her. 'I know you said to Amara that your back was fixed, but isn't it going to be tough for you to face heights again?'

'Abseiling is a completely different situation from doing a roof inspection,' he said. 'Yes, it scares me, but it'll do me good to face that last, lingering fear.' He paused. 'So have you had a bad experience with heights, then?'

'No. I'm just aware of the risks.' The sort of risks Lucas had taken. The sort of risks that had literally made him crash. 'The idea of just one little rope being between me and a huge drop... That makes my palms sweat.'

'You'd be on a safety line and you really couldn't fall,' he said. 'I know what you mean about sweaty palms. I'm scared, too. But I weighed up the risks before I said yes. And we need that scanner. So the way I see it is you have to ignore the scary stuff and just get it done.'

Ignore the scary stuff and just get it done. Which wasn't the same as being a risk-chaser. It was about being confident, not over-confident and cocky. Taking calculated risks. Ignoring the voice in your head that made you miss out on things. And that confidence drew her even more. 'That's pretty good advice for life in general,' she said thoughtfully.

His eyes were kind as he said, 'Sometimes it's easy to overthink things.'

Since Lucas, she knew that she had a tendency to do that. Maybe she should take Nathaniel's advice. Be brave. Ask him out. Her skin suddenly felt a bit too tight, but she ignored it. What was the worst that could happen? If he said no, she'd back off. And if he said yes... Actually, she wasn't going to think about that, because it was even scarier.

'You're right. Sometimes it's easy to overthink things. And sometimes you think about it again afterwards and realise it should've been simple. Like—' She took a deep breath to steady her nerves. 'Like going out for a pizza with someone.'

That got his attention. He met her gaze head-on, and his dark eyes were warm and sweet, with a hint of sultriness. 'A pizza.'

Stop overthinking it, she told herself. *What does it matter that you haven't dated anyone except Lucas for six and a half years? What does it matter that you've never asked someone out before? This is a simple yes-or-no question. A first step. Do it.*

'Uh-huh.' She cleared her throat again. 'That pizza you suggested last week. Would you—are you—could we—?' Oh, for pity's sake. Since when was she so inarticulate? Keep it simple. 'Could we do it?'

The corner of his mouth quirked. 'That sounded like a proposition, Dr Hart.'

She felt the colour flood through her face. 'It…' she croaked.

His grin broadened. 'Sorry. I was teasing you. It was irresistible. Of course I know you were talking about pizza.'

Though he'd made it sound like sex.

He'd made her think of sex.

He'd made her think of things she'd shut down for years. She couldn't speak, just nodded.

'I'd love to have pizza with you.' He paused. 'Are we talking as a team thing?'

She shook her head. 'Just…'

'Good friends?'

She dragged in a breath. 'I haven't dated anyone since Lucas died. I've never asked anyone out. I'm…' She shook her head. 'I don't know how to do this.'

'But you *did* do it. You've thought about it; you ignored the scary bit and did it,' he said. 'And, yes, I'd like to go out with you. Very much. Which isn't something I'm used to feeling, either.'

Funny how that made her feel better; though at the same time she wondered why someone as nice and as gorgeous as Nathaniel Jones was single. Had someone broken his heart? 'OK. When's good for you?'

'I can be flexible.' He paused. 'What about you? Would an evening be a problem?'

'No. My mum or my sister will be happy to babysit.' She smiled wryly. 'Actually, my sister will be thrilled as she's been nagging me for ages to date again.'

'I know how that feels,' he said. 'My big sister is always on my case.'

'Little ones can nag just as much, believe me,' she said feelingly.

So they'd both been nagged to date someone.

And their pizza—even though it would be low-key and casual—was going to be a proper date. The fact made her feel ridiculously shy, as if she were a teenager all over again. Considering she was the one who'd asked him out, the shyness was even more ridiculous. She got a grip on herself. Just. 'Are you free on Monday evening?'

He took his phone from his pocket and checked his diary. 'Monday evening's fine.'

'OK. I'll book a table and text you the details.'

'What's your number?' he asked. 'Then I'll text you so you've got my number.'

She recited it, and a couple of moments later her phone pinged with a message from him.

And that was it.

They were officially going on a date.

And, instead of being scared by it, she found that it made the world feel weirdly brighter. It made *her* feel brighter, too. Encouraged. Empowered.

'All right,' she said. 'I'll do the abseil.'

'You really don't have to. I can find someone else,' he said.

'No, you're right. Of course it's safe. The people who set things up do that every day. They do a ton of checks.'

'And think about it this way: they'd be terrified at the idea of delivering a baby, which you do without batting an eyelid,' he said.

'I guess. OK. And my daughter won't have to see it. She has a swimming lesson in the morning—Mum was going with me, but Dad can go in my place.'

'Aren't you going to have anyone with you to cheer you on?' he asked. 'I'm bringing my sister and her wife.'

'I could ask my sister,' Rebecca said.

'Thank you. Though I meant it about no pressure.' He gave her another of those smiles that made her heart flip. 'Excuse the pun—no strings.'

'I definitely don't want strings. I want nice, solid ropes.' That was how she'd wanted her relationship to be, too. Strong and solid. But the supports had turned out to be flimsy. She shook herself. 'But you were right. I need to face the fear.' She didn't want Jasmine to grow up being a thrill-seeker like her dad; but she was starting to think that going too far the other way and wrapping her in cotton wool would cause just as many problems. Doing something that scared her, in a safe environment, was a good way to help her find the right balance.

The rest of the day flew by; Rebecca booked the table, that evening, and texted the details to Nathaniel.

Meet you there at seven.

He texted back.

Looking forward to it.

So was she.

But they had the abseil to get through, first. Friday went by incredibly quickly.

And then on Saturday morning she met Nathaniel, along with the rest of the team, in the centre of London. Between them they had quite a throng of supporters, all armed with cameras.

'Saskia, this is my colleague Nathaniel, who's just joined our team. Nathaniel, this is my sister, Saskia,' she introduced them swiftly.

'Delighted to meet you,' he said, shaking her hand. 'And this is my sister, Charlotte, and her wife, Robyn,' Nathaniel said, indicating a heavily pregnant woman who looked so much like him that even without the introduction Rebecca would've guessed that was his sister, and a slender woman with a kind smile. 'Guys, meet some of my new team.' He introduced his family to everyone on the Muswell Hill Memorial Hospital's team. 'I guess we'll see you all back here at the bottom.'

'Good luck, Bec!' Saskia said.

And then Rebecca was heading for the top of the building with the rest of the team, to have her harness and helmet fitted. She and Nathaniel were the first two to walk along the metal openwork pathway next to the security fence. Suddenly it felt a very, very long way up. Even the tops of the tallest buildings across the city seemed a long way below them.

Why on earth had she ever thought that this was a good idea? Had she been temporarily insane when she'd agreed to join the team abseil?

Obviously her fear showed in her face, because Nathaniel asked softly, 'Are you OK?'

No. She was incredibly nervous and even the

thought of what she was about to do made her hands feel sweaty. 'Fine,' she fibbed. 'You?'

'Fine.'

The calmness in his voice and his smile made her feel very slightly better.

'It's going to be OK,' he said. 'There are lots and lots and *lots* of layers of security. It's safe, or they wouldn't let you do it. We're not the first team to go down today.'

No, but they were the first of *their* team.

'You've got this,' he said. 'I've seen you in Theatre performing a C-section. If you can deliver a baby and sew all those layers of muscle and skin back together in that short a time, and so neatly, then you can do this one tiny little abseil. Ten minutes, that's all it'll take. You can do *anything* for ten minutes, Rebecca. Anything at all. And that's all this will take. Ten minutes. You've got this.'

If this was how he talked his mums through contractions and breathing, no wonder he was so popular on the ward, she thought. He was calm and reassuring, and—more importantly—she believed what he was telling her.

She trusted him.

'OK,' she said.

Though her nerves came back when she stepped up onto the platform and the woman from the event team clipped her carabiner and safety rope on. She was vaguely aware of Nathaniel standing next to her, going through the same safety checks, but she was even more aware of the open space behind her. The sheer drop. And she was going to have to walk backwards over the edge…

'Now your gloves. They're thick enough to handle the rope and protect your hands,' the woman said. 'I'll talk you through it.'

Rebecca could feel clamminess on her face and the racing of her heart. 'OK,' she said.

'I want you to go to the outer edge and hold on to the bar. You're not going to fall, and you'll be perfectly safe,' the instructor reassured her.

Every step felt as if her feet were made of lead. She was shuffling rather than picking her feet up.

'Now put both your hands on the rope.'

'Let go of the bar?' Her voice sounded as quivery as it felt.

'You're clipped on. You won't fall,' the woman told her. 'Both hands on the rope, lean back, and keep your shoulders back—it should feel like you're sitting down, but your legs are out straight instead of bent.'

Her movements felt slow, as if they were going through treacle, but finally Rebecca managed it.

'Now lift the rope up. It'll feel heavy to start with, but it gets easier.'

It definitely felt heavy.

'As you go down, the rope will be lighter so you'll go faster. But you're in control of your speed,' the instructor continued. 'When you push the rope up through your hands, you'll start to go down. Take your time. There's no rush.'

No, but she was dithering so much that she was holding everyone else up. She glanced to the side, expecting that Nathaniel would be long gone—but, to her surprise, he was there, waiting for her.

'Hey. I thought we could do this together,' he said.

'OK.' She was aware that she was talking through clenched teeth. How could he be this calm and sanguine, all this distance up?

'Rebecca? I want you to start going backwards now. One foot at a time. You'll feel a ledge beneath your feet,' the instructor said.

Slowly, slowly, she got her feet to move. The rope's weight made her arms ache.

'Spread your toes to keep your balance, and take another step,' the instructor said. 'Over the ledge. You can do it. Remember there are people waiting for you at the bottom to help you, and you're not going to fall because we've got you. Take your time, enjoy the views, and think of all the money you're raising.'

One step. Over the ledge.

Rebecca was terrified, but she made herself do it.

Then there was a clicking sound that made her panic. 'What's that?' she asked. 'It's clicking. Does that mean something's going wrong?' Her blood was roaring in her ears.

'It's just the rope going through the pulley. The clicks mean it's working and you're safe,' Nathaniel said. 'Come on. One step at a time. Down we go. Wave to your sister. Make her proud of you.'

She managed it. Just. Then she made the mistake of looking down. And it was a long way down. A long, long, *long* way to fall. Why had she ever thought that this was a good idea? Why hadn't she just said no? 'Oh, my God.'

'Don't look down,' he said. 'Look across to me. See me smiling at you.'

He was smiling, all the way up here, even though he'd fallen off a roof and broken his back. And that confidence warmed her. Boosted her. Nathaniel Jones was amazing. He'd hurt himself—very badly—yet here he was, up here with her, facing his fears and raising money for the ward.

If he could do this without shaking, so could

she. Because he knew what it was like to fall from up high, what the crunching of bones sounded like, what the shock of impact felt like.

'One more step,' he encouraged. 'Take a little step, and push that rope up. You just have to travel one hundred times your height, and then you'll be back with your feet on the ground.'

A hundred times her own height hadn't sounded so bad, on the ground. Now she was actually up here, it was terrifying.

'You're doing great,' he said. Just as if he were encouraging one of his mums through a contraction. 'You've got this. Baby steps. Down we go. Push that rope up.'

And, gradually, the earth began to move a bit closer.

Down they went.

'Look at me,' he said.

She did so. How warm and sweet and soulful his brown eyes were. How beautiful his mouth was. Why hadn't she noticed in the time they'd been working together? Nathaniel Jones was every bit as gorgeous as a heart-throb movie actor, and she wanted to look at him a lot more than she wanted to look at the view.

'You can do this. Keep going. Push that rope and take another step,' he encouraged.

Just as the instructor had said, the rope gradually felt lighter and lighter. And either she really was going faster, or she felt a bit less scared than she had at the top, because suddenly they were whizzing down and she was actually enjoying it—to the point where she could risk looking out, and the city looked beautiful instead of much too far away. Finally, she understood why people liked an adrenalin rush. Right at that moment, she felt as if she could conquer the world.

She glanced across at Nathaniel. Just then, it felt as if there were only the two of them, suspended in space. Floating.

Was this how it would feel if she danced with him? As if she were walking on air, weightless?

He was looking right back at her, and there was a bloom of colour in his cheeks. Was he thinking the same thing? she wondered. Thinking about how it would feel to be in each other's arms, their mouths just a touch apart, on the brink of a kiss?

For a second, she couldn't breathe.

'OK?' he asked.

Yes. No. She didn't have a clue. 'I feel…' She shook her head, unable to articulate it. 'This whole thing…'

'It's pretty amazing,' he said, his voice husky.

So was he. Again, her breath caught. 'You're pretty amazing,' she blurted out.

'Takes one to know one,' he said, and her

heart skipped a beat. Was he saying he thought she was amazing, too?

'Let's finish this,' he said. 'You're doing brilliantly. Wave to your sister and smile.'

And this time she could look down. She could see Saskia standing there on the ground at the front of the spectators, waving madly.

She waved back and grinned.

'Well done. Keep going,' he said.

Down they went, step by step, the rope clicking, until finally they were at the bottom; there were people helping her touch down and unclipping her from the ropes. Nathaniel was standing next to her, having just taken off his hard hat, gloves and harness.

'We did it.' She flung her arms round him and held him close. 'Thank you. If you hadn't talked me down...'

'You would still have done it,' he said. Though he was holding her just as tightly, as if he didn't want to let go of her either.

She looked him straight in the eye. Suspended in mid-air, she'd thought his eyes were dark and soulful. Close up, she could see that there were little flecks of gold and green in his dark brown eyes. Like little bits of sunlight. And his mouth was beautifully shaped, only a few centimetres from her own; his lips were slightly parted. She felt her own lips parting, felt herself rising up on her toes ready to touch her mouth to his.

And the rush she felt when their lips met was even stronger than the rush she'd felt as she'd abseiled down the building. Here, with Nathaniel kissing her, the rest of the world fell away. It felt as if they were alone on the top of a cliff with the sun shining down and the sea lapping against the sand, far below.

Except it wasn't lapping.

It was *clapping*.

She opened her eyes in shock and pulled back.

Dear God. She'd snogged the face off Nathaniel Jones in front of her sister and quite a few of her department. And now everyone was *clapping*. How were they ever going to live this down?

She risked a glance at Nathaniel.

Those gorgeous eyes still had those green and golden flecks—but he looked slightly dazed, as if she hadn't been the only one carried away by the rush of the abseil.

Except it wasn't the abseil. It was *Nathaniel* who'd made her feel this rush, this thrill of pleasure. That kiss. The feel of his heart thudding against hers. The warmth of his body.

What was she going to do?

What was *he* going to do?

She didn't have a clue. She had no idea what to do, what to say, what to...

He recovered first. 'It's so long since I did anything like abseiling, I'd forgotten what a buzz it gives you. I think my last lingering fear of falling might just be over. Thank you for sharing the moment, Dr Hart, and I apologise for getting carried away.'

He was going to take the blame?

Gallant, but she couldn't quite let him do that, it wasn't fair. She'd been the one to instigate it. 'And I think my fear of heights might be cured, too. You're right. It's easy to get carried away—and I apologise, too, Mr Jones.'

Please don't let anyone work out that she was lying though her teeth.

That kiss might have started out from relief at being back on solid ground, but it definitely hadn't ended that way. The end of that kiss had been about desire, pure and simple.

And she hadn't been alone. He'd kissed her back.

'I, um—I need to go and collect my daughter,' she said.

'And I think we both need to reassure our sisters,' he said.

'I...um—see you Monday.' And she fled before she could say or do anything else stupid.

Though of course Saskia had seen everything.

'I assume that was the guy you're seeing on Monday night when I'm babysitting?' she asked, fanning herself. 'Whoa. Mr Darcy, eat your heart out. I think any woman would want to snog him.'

Rebecca groaned. 'Sas. Please don't tease. I feel… Oh, my God. I snogged him in front of everyone.' She put her hands to her face in horror. 'How am I going to face the rumour mill at work on Monday?'

'Just tell them it was the adrenalin rush from the abseil,' Saskia suggested.

'We already did.'

'Good. You've probably nipped it in the bud. If you haven't, then just brazen it out and make them give you extra money for sponsorship.' Saskia raised an eyebrow. 'I haven't seen you look this flustered since you were a teenager.'

'I don't think I've *felt* this flustered since I was a teenager,' Rebecca admitted. Except maybe in the early days with Lucas, but she hadn't had any responsibilities to worry about back then. Now, she did. She couldn't afford to be flustered.

'It'll do you good to be flustered,' Saskia said. 'You need some fun.'

Fun? Rebecca wasn't quite sure this was fun. It was scary. Nathaniel was the first man she'd dated since Lucas. The first man in years who'd put her in a spin. And she didn't know whether that was going to be a good thing or a bad.

Later that evening, once Jasmine was asleep, Rebecca was about to text Nathaniel to thank him for talking her through the abseil when her phone beeped with an incoming message.

You were very brave today.

She typed back, wanting to be honest,

I was very scared. Thank you for talking me down.

And they were going to have to talk about what had happened afterwards.

Sorry for...

Except she wasn't sorry for kissing him. Not in the slightest.

Sorry if I've made it awkward at work.

He texted back,

We both got carried away by the rush of the moment.

Meaning that the kiss hadn't affected him and she was setting herself up for disappointment already?

Her phone beeped again.

At least, that's all they need to know.

Meaning that kiss *had* affected him the same way that it had affected her. Feeling better, she texted.

Looking forward to Monday.

She added a kiss and sent it.

She didn't have to wait long for an answer.

So am I. x

That kiss at the end made her feel like a teenager all over again, fluttery and excited.

Monday was going to be...

Fun, she reminded herself. *Keep it light. Enjoy it instead of worrying.*

CHAPTER FIVE

WHAT DID YOU wear for a first date? Jeans were a bit too casual, Rebecca thought; on the other hand, a little black dress would be a bit over the top, given that they were only going to the local pizzeria. She didn't want to seem too keen, but she also didn't want to look as if she hadn't made any effort. In the end, she settled for a pretty summer dress and wore her hair loose.

Her sister, who adored Jasmine, was babysitting, and Rebecca was relaxed as she walked out of her front door; but her nerves kicked in with every step she took towards the restaurant and by the time she reached the pizzeria her fingers were tingling with adrenalin. Was she doing the right thing? Was she really ready to date again? Why did even the prospect of dating Nathaniel make her feel all at sixes and sevens?

This was simply having a casual dinner together in a restaurant she knew well; there shouldn't be anything intimidating about it. Yet it was hard to make herself open the door.

Nathaniel was already there when she walked into the restaurant and confirmed that she had a table booked. He stood up when she reached him, and she rather liked his old-fashioned manners.

'Hi,' she said.

'Thanks for coming,' he said, smiling. 'You look lovely.'

'Thanks. So do you,' she added shyly. He was wearing a smart-casual burgundy shirt and dark trousers, teamed with suede shoes—very different from the navy scrubs he wore on the ward. Here, he wasn't a midwife, another member of her team on the ward: he was a man. The man she'd kissed after the abseil. *The man she was starting to date.* And she wasn't sure if that made her more scared or thrilled.

'What would you like to drink?' he asked.

'A glass of red wine would be nice,' she said.

'I'll join you. Shall we order a bottle?'

'Sure.'

'Chianti OK with you?' he checked.

'That'd be lovely.'

Once they'd ordered their wine and pizzas, with salad and dough balls to share, Rebecca's nerves flickered again. It was so long since she'd dated that she'd forgotten the etiquette.

Why on earth hadn't she looked up some tips on the internet, first? Her social skills seemed to have deserted her entirely.

At least work would be a safe topic of conversation. 'How was your day?' she asked.

'Brilliant. I had a first-time mum in, everything went almost completely according to her birth plan, and the dad cut the cord and bawled his eyes out.' He grinned. 'I love days like this. How about you?'

'I did a section,' she said, 'after the poor mum had been in labour all night. She was gutted, but the baby was starting to show signs of distress and she was exhausted.'

'You did the right thing, then.'

'Yes.'

Silence spun between them. Oh, help. Had they exhausted work as a topic? What now? She was about to make an anodyne comment about the weather when he surprised her by asking, 'What made you change your mind about going on a date with me?'

Because she couldn't get him out of her head. Not that she wanted to admit that. Not yet. 'It was time I started dating again,' she said instead. Though she knew she needed to tell him about what had happened to Lucas. 'Just so it doesn't become the elephant in the room, I'd better explain about my husband. He was a doctor in the emergency department, and...' She paused. 'Let's just say Lucas liked an adrenalin rush. He used to ride a motorbike. One night, he hit a patch of ice and crashed. Nobody else was involved, but he didn't survive the accident.'

'I'm sorry,' he said. 'That must have been hard for you.'

'It was.'

'How old was Jasmine when he was killed?' Nathaniel asked.

'Just over a year.' She bit her lip. They'd been dark days indeed. And she'd been so grateful for her family's support.

Losing her husband in a crash, when their daughter was only a year old. Rebecca would've had to be strong for the little girl, rather than letting herself grieve. No wonder she didn't date, Nathaniel thought.

'I'm sorry,' he said again.

For both their sakes, he should stop this now. Tip it back over the line into friendship.

The problem was, he didn't want to.

She was the first woman who'd intrigued him this much since Angela. He really wanted to know where this could go.

He didn't want to explain about Angela, because he didn't want Rebecca to pity him. But maybe there was a middle ground. She'd mentioned that Lucas had been an adrenalin junkie; Nathaniel could at least assuage that fear.

'Just so you know, despite the fact I fell off a roof and I was OK about doing the abseiling on Saturday, I'm not a thrill seeker. But I haven't been in a serious relationship for a while.'

'You've been busy changing careers,' she said. 'There isn't much time for fun when you're juggling shifts and lectures and everything else.'

It was technically true; just nowhere near the whole truth. But it was enough for now. So he smiled and said, 'Yes.'

She spread her hands. 'I'm so rusty when it comes to dating. I'm totally clueless about etiquette.'

He rather liked the way she'd admitted that. And the way she wrinkled her nose was oh, so cute.

'What are we even supposed to talk about?' she asked.

'On our first date? I guess we'd talk about what we do for a living, and then what sort of things we like,' he said. 'You and I already know about each other's work. So I'll start the next topic: are you a dog person or a cat person?'

'Neither,' she said. 'I'd love a dog, but I don't

have one because it wouldn't be fair when I'm not home very much. You?'

'Cat. I have a Bengal cat called Leo—because he looks like a mini leopard.'

'Seriously?'

'Seriously.' He took his phone from his pocket and flicked into the photographs before handing the phone to her. 'Here you go.'

'Oh—he's very pretty,' she said, sounding surprised. 'He really does look like a mini leopard.'

'And he's a total sweetheart. He kind of thinks he's a dog, so he'll sit or he'll do a high-five if you ask him to,' Nathaniel said with a grin. 'He's ten, now. And he kept me sane when I was recovering from the accident. He stayed right by my side. And he used to miaow when I was doing physio, almost as if he was telling me to keep going. As if he was counting the reps for me.'

'That's really cute.' She smiled and handed the phone back.

'OK. What kind of music do you like?'

'Anything I can sing to, but I guess I like the eighties stuff my parents used to play when I was a kid,' she said. 'You?'

'Classic rock. That's my dad's influence. He used to play in a band.' He thought about it. 'Best film ever?'

'*It's a Wonderful Life*,' she said promptly. 'Followed very closely by *Love, Actually*.'

Interesting choice. Films with a bit of darkness but a lot of happiness. Was that what she was looking for—the happiness after the darkness she'd had to endure so young? 'So you're a Christmas fan?'

'It's purely coincidental that they're both Christmas films. It's the happy endings I like,' she said.

She wanted a happy ending.

This was their first date. He couldn't guarantee anything. But he'd do his best to make today happy for her.

'How about you? What are your favourite films?' she asked.

'*The Empire Strikes Back*,' he said. 'Followed by *Raiders of the Lost Ark*.'

She smiled. 'I'm guessing that's influenced by your dad, again?'

'Absolutely.' He spread his hands. 'Do you prefer sea or mountains?'

'Sea,' she said promptly.

'Me, too. Cheese or chocolate?'

'Cheese.'

'Chocolate,' he said. 'Which is also the answer to what's the best ice cream ever.'

'No, that's salted caramel,' she said. 'Favourite food?'

'Jamaican,' he said. 'My best friend's parents are from Jamaica. His mum makes the most amazing run-down stew.'

'Run-down stew? What's that?'

'Fish,' he said, 'stewed with coconut milk, tomatoes and spices until it falls apart. Served with dumplings. Her fried dumplings are like nothing you've ever tasted. They're amazing.' Bits of him knew he ought to shut up now, but his mouth wasn't running with the programme. 'Actually, Rita taught me how to cook them. So maybe—if you decide you'd like a second date with me—I can cook stew and dumplings for you. Leo will be pleased, because it'll mean he gets fish.'

Part of Rebecca loved the idea of a man who could handle domestic stuff—someone who could cook, instead of forgetting to order take-out and leaving everything to her. But part of her worried. Eating dinner at his place would be much, much more intimate than eating in a crowded restaurant. It was too big a step for her to take right now. 'I…can we take a rain check on that?' she asked, biting her lip and feeling awkward.

A rain check.

Nathaniel realised he'd tried to take this too

fast. Their food hadn't even arrived yet, and he was asking her for a second date? Ridiculous. No wonder she'd backed off. Time to keep things light.

Except the little insidious voice in the back of his head—the one that had plagued him in his hospital bed, after Angie had dumped him—whispered, *She's just trying to be polite. Why would a successful, clever, beautiful woman like her want to date you? She's out of your league and there's no way you'll be enough for her—just like you weren't enough for Angie.*

He took a sip of wine to distract himself. He'd silenced that voice of doubt before and he'd do it again. Technically, Rebecca had asked him out. Which she wouldn't have done if she was simply being polite. This was a first date, and first dates were always awkward.

'Sure,' he said, trying to be kind and not let her guess how horrible he felt right then.

Their pizzas arrived then, and he kept the conversation light—about books, favourite holidays, and cake.

And then her fingers accidentally brushed against his as they reached for a dough ball at the same time. It felt as if he'd been galvanised. And, when he looked at her, he could see it was the same for her.

'Sorry,' she muttered. 'I...'

He guessed that she was finding this as awkward as he was. Her situation made dating a minefield.

'Me, too,' he said. 'This dating thing is hard, particularly when you're a single parent. I'm not going to push you into doing anything you're not ready for.'

'Thank you.' She looked relieved, and he had to suppress another whisper of insecurity.

'Perhaps we can be kind to each other,' he said. 'See where this takes us.'

Be kind? That sounded as if someone had been less than kind to him. Had someone broken his heart? Rebecca wondered. Though asking felt too intrusive, right now. And she was grateful that he was being understanding rather than pushy.

'Being kind sounds perfect to me,' she said.

When they'd finished their pizzas, they lingered for a coffee, and then Nathaniel suggested walking her home. 'The long way round. Via the park—I haven't had time to explore much, since I moved here, but it looks nice.'

'It is,' she said. 'Whether it's all the blossom on the trees in spring, or the roses in summer, or the trees in autumn—actually, it's even nice in winter. And Jas loves it there. I'm sure your goddaughter would, too.'

'Perfect for kids to run around. Do you have a garden?'

She nodded.

'You're lucky. My flat has space for a couple of pots of herbs on the kitchen windowsill, and that's it.'

He grew herbs on his windowsill? 'So you like cooking?'

'I found it relaxed me after a day at work, when I was still in the building trade,' he said. 'And then, when I was stuck in bed and waiting to see if I could walk again, looking at recipes and planning how I was going to tweak them was one of the things that kept me sane. There's only so much sport I could stand watching on TV.'

'I'll bet. It must've been really hard for you.'

'I got through it.' He shrugged. 'The only other choice was to give up.'

And he clearly wasn't the sort to give up easily, or he wouldn't have got back to walking again and then switching careers completely. 'I guess,' she said.

As they walked through the park, his hand brushed against hers a couple of times, sending tingles through her. The third time, he let his fingers curl round hers; it wasn't demanding or a gesture of possession, but gave her more of a sense of promise.

The more she was getting to know Nathaniel, the more she liked him. He was sweet, funny and romantic. And walking hand in hand through the park with him made her feel like a teenager again—though carefree and light of heart, rather than socially awkward.

She remembered that moment after the abseil when she'd kissed him. How she'd forgotten everything and everyone around them, only aware of the feel of his mouth against hers and the way her blood had surged through her veins.

Would he kiss her tonight?

Would it make her have that floaty feeling all over again?

Anticipation tingled through her as they reached her gate.

'My sister's babysitting,' she said.

'If it was my sister babysitting,' he said, 'she'd start grilling you the second you walked through the door.'

'Saskia is a psychologist,' she said. 'So, yes. There would be grilling.' She had to be honest. 'Professional-level grilling. So I know it's rude not to invite you in for coffee, but…'

'It's fine. I understand. Goodnight, Rebecca. And thank you for a lovely evening.'

So he wasn't going to kiss her. He'd said earlier that he wouldn't be pushy. She liked the fact that he'd kept his word; though, at the same time, part of her was disappointed. Because she'd been itching to kiss Nathaniel Jones again ever since he'd taken her hand in the park. She'd wanted to feel like a carefree teenager again. 'Goodnight, Nathaniel. And thank you for seeing me home.'

He was still holding her hand. 'I'd really like to kiss you goodnight,' he said, his voice as soft and smooth as melted chocolate. 'But that's going to be your choice.'

The heat in his eyes made her knees weak.

'Yes,' she said.

'Good,' he said, and dipped his head.

It was a sweet, gossamer-light kiss, brushing her lips just enough to make them tingle. A kiss full of promise—a promise that next time the warmth would scorch into flame. Just as it had after the abseil, making her head spin and the rest of the world vanish.

'Goodnight, sweet Rebecca,' he whispered.

'Goodnight.' Her voice sounded as wobbly as her knees felt.

'I'll wait here until you're safely inside. See you at work,' he said.

Despite her wobbly knees, she managed to walk to her front door without tripping over, then turned to wave at him. He lifted his hand in acknowledgement, then turned away.

She opened the front door with a smile on her face. This evening had been a revelation. With Nathaniel, her spirit felt so light, not weighed down with worry. Yet, at the same time, she had the feeling that he understood the fact that she had responsibilities; he was taking things at a pace that suited her, rather than rushing her the way Lucas had.

Later that evening, Rebecca's phone beeped with a text from Nathaniel.

Really enjoyed this evening. Thank you. See you tomorrow. N x

I enjoyed it too. R x

On impulse, she added,

So what wine do I bring to go with fish stew and dumplings?

Then she panicked and deleted it, replacing it with,

See you tomorrow. x

He sent a smiley face back.
She couldn't remember the last time she'd felt

quite this light of heart. Her lips tingled as she thought about that kiss, so sweet and so full of promise. And she really, really wanted him to kiss her again.

The next morning, when Rebecca did the ward rounds, she really wasn't happy about Josette Kamanya's blood pressure. She sat down next to her and took her hand. 'Despite the medication, your blood pressure still isn't down enough for my liking, Mrs Kamanya. I think we've got to the point where we need to deliver your baby to keep you both safe.'

Mrs Kamanya's eyes widened. 'I'm only thirty-five weeks. Surely it's still too soon?'

'If it makes you feel any better,' Rebecca said gently, 'around eight per cent are born before thirty-seven weeks. I'd like to give you steroids to mature the baby's lungs, and give you a section tomorrow. Your husband can still be there during the delivery, holding your hand, and he can still cut the cord, so your birth plan isn't *completely* out of the window.'

'But what happens then?' Mrs Kamanya looked pinched with fear.

'We'll have someone from the neonatal team in with us during your delivery, and they'll take the baby in to the Special Care Baby Unit at first, just while he or she needs a bit of extra help feeding, breathing and staying warm. Then, when the baby's ready, they'll move him or her to the neonatal unit.'

A tear rolled down Mrs Kamanya's face, and Rebecca squeezed her hand. 'I know it's not what you wanted, and I'm sorry about that, but I promise you it's going to be fine. You'll still be able to feed the baby yourself and you'll still be able to do a lot of the care. It really won't make a huge difference that the baby's a little bit early.'

Just then, Nathaniel walked through the ward and came over to them.

'Good morning,' Rebecca said.

'Morning,' he replied, smiling.

The heat in his eyes made her pulse skitter, and she had to take a deep breath to tamp it down. Right now Mrs Kamanya needed her to be professional, not distracted by her emotions.

'I can see that everything's not OK. How are you doing, Mrs Kamanya?' he asked.

Her voice wobbled. 'Dr Hart says we need to deliver the baby tomorrow.'

Nathaniel sat on the opposite side of the bed to Rebecca and took Mrs Kamanya's other hand. 'To keep the baby safe, because your blood pressure's still higher than we'd like it to be. But I can tell you I've seen Rebecca operate, and she's *magic*.'

'I just wanted everything to...' Mrs Kamanya dragged in a breath. 'To go like I planned it.'

A natural birth, with just gas and air—the thing most of their first-time mums wanted. And most of them ended up screwing their birth plan into a ball and throwing it in the bin. 'Babies are notorious for disrespecting birth plans,' Rebecca said. 'I'm not sure I know anyone who actually had the kind of delivery they planned—and that includes me.'

'You?' Mrs Kamanya looked surprised.

'Absolutely. As an obstetrician, I should've known better, but I hadn't quite finished packing my labour bag when my daughter decided she was ready to come into the world,' Rebecca admitted. 'Jasmine was two weeks early—and she's nearly five now and bright as a button.'

'The same thing happened with my goddaughter,' Nathaniel said. 'She's four. Sienna decided to be born while her dad—my best friend—was on a business trip in Scotland. Denise went into labour early and I ended up being her stand-by birth partner. I fell in love with seeing babies delivered, and that's why I became a midwife. I love those first moments after a baby's arrived into the world—they're really special.'

Rebecca rather thought that Nathaniel might be special, too, but didn't voice it aloud. 'I agree. Those first moments are so precious. I remember every single baby I've ever delivered, and I never get tired of newborn cuddles.'

Mrs Kamanya gave them both a wobbly smile. 'So what happens now?'

'What we'll do today is give you two steroid injections, twelve hours apart, to mature the baby's lungs,' Rebecca said. 'Then we'll deliver the baby tomorrow morning.' She squeezed Mrs Kamanya's hand again. 'So the good news is, you're not going to be like the mums who are hot and tired in the middle of summer and wishing their baby wasn't nearly two weeks late. You'll be able to see your baby tomorrow.'

Mrs Kamanya bit her lip. 'But if the baby's in Special Care, doesn't that mean I won't be able to hold the baby or do anything?'

'You can hold the baby and do lots of things,' Nathaniel said. 'Though your baby will look a bit different from what you'd expect from a newborn. He or she'll look a bit thinner, the skin will be quite red and maybe there'll be a bit of down on the baby's face, though that'll change quickly as the baby grows.'

'The baby will be in an incubator at first,' Rebecca said, 'but you'll soon be able to do what we call "kangaroo care". If you wear a front-opening top and dress the baby in a nappy and a hat, you can hold the baby against your chest and wrap your top round you both. You'll be skin to skin, which helps your baby maintain a healthy body temperature and also helps you and the baby to bond.'

'What if they need to put tubes and wires on the baby?' Mrs Kamanya asked.

'You can still do the kangaroo care,' Nathaniel said, 'but you just need to stay near the machines. And you can stroke the baby, make eye contact, talk and sing to the baby, and the baby can hold your finger, just as if your baby was full-term.'

'You might be able to breastfeed the baby, too, if that was what you'd planned,' Rebecca added. 'The nurses can help you, though if the baby can't quite latch on you can still express milk so you can feed the baby through a tube from her nose to her stomach.'

'Do you want us to call someone to be with you today?' Nathaniel asked.

Mrs Kamanya nodded. 'I really want Andras here.'

'I'll go and call him now,' Rebecca promised, 'and I'll come back to let you know when he'll be here.'

'And I'll stay with you for a little while—my clinic doesn't start for another ten minutes,' Nathaniel said.

* * *

After his clinic, Nathaniel was in the staff kitchen, making coffee, when Rebecca walked in.

'Perfect timing. Coffee?' he asked.

'Love one, please. Though I've got about three minutes to drink it,' she warned. 'My clinic was running late this morning, and I'm in Theatre this afternoon.'

'I'm on it.' He dissolved the coffee in boiling water, added milk, then added cold water so she could drink it straight down.

'Thank you. You have no idea how much I appreciate that,' she said.

Funny how her smile made his heart skip a beat. The warmth, the sweetness... And his mouth tingled as he remembered kissing her, the previous night.

He wanted to kiss her again, but here in the staff kitchen really wasn't the right place. Besides, he wasn't entirely sure how she felt about it. She'd texted him to say she'd had a lovely evening—but she hadn't said anything about a second date.

Play it cool, he told himself. *Take it slowly.*

'How's your morning been?' he asked.

'Good. Yours?'

'Good. Actually, I need to catch you up on one of our mums. Mrs Ridley was in clinic this morning.' He smiled. 'You'll be pleased to know the baby hasn't decided to turn back the other way and his head's nicely engaged in her pelvis.'

'That's great news,' Rebecca said with a smile. 'So she's thirty-seven weeks, now. Hopefully we'll see her in a couple of weeks and it'll be a nice easy delivery, to make up for all that discomfort.'

'They've got their labour bag packed, and Matt's done a test run several times so he knows exactly how long it takes to get here.'

She laughed. 'Bless. It's lovely when the dads get really involved.'

Was it his imagination, or was there a faint bit of wistfulness in her eyes? She hadn't said much about her marriage, but she'd mentioned that Lucas was an adrenalin junkie. In his experience, that didn't go well with the demands of a baby. Had her husband maybe not supported her during her pregnancy and when Jasmine was tiny?

It was none of his business, and it would be way too intrusive to ask. Better to keep everything impersonal and work-related. 'Yeah. It's lovely when the dads are really part of it,' he agreed.

'Righty—it's off to Theatre for me. Catch you later. And thanks for the coffee,' she said.

'Pleasure. Catch you later,' he said.

* * *

Rebecca administered the second dose of steroids on the Tuesday evening, and Mrs Kamanya was her first mum due in Theatre on Wednesday morning. Mrs Kamanya's husband, Andras, was there to hold her hand; Rebecca introduced them both to the anaesthetist, who took them through consent for the operation, and she explained exactly what was going to happen. Then she went to scrub in and prep for Theatre; she was pleased to see that Nathaniel was on the team.

The operation went smoothly, Mr Kamanya cut the cord, and Nathaniel was there to check the Apgar score once the baby was delivered.

'I'm pleased to say you have a healthy little girl,' he said. 'She weighs two and a quarter kilograms, and she's forty centimetres long, so she's doing very nicely.'

Both parents had happy tears running down their cheeks.

'Can we hold her for a minute?' Mr Kamanya asked.

'Of course, but then she's going off to Special Care to warm up.' Nathaniel handed the baby, wrapped in a blanket, to Mr Kamanya.

'Our precious little girl,' he whispered. 'Look, Jose. She's perfect.'

'Our precious little girl,' Mrs Kamanya echoed.

Rebecca could see moisture in Nathaniel's eyes when he took the baby back, ready to hand her over to the neonatal team. He really cared, she thought. And he had a proper emotional connection with their mums, which made him good to work with.

She finished sewing Mrs Kamanya back up. 'We'll keep you in the recovery room next door for about half an hour, just to keep an eye on you and make sure everything's as it should be, then we'll sort out a wheelchair and get you to the Special Care Baby Unit so you can be with your little girl,' she said. 'You're doing really well. Have you decided on a name, yet?'

'Kayleigh,' Mrs Kamanya said.

'That's a lovely name,' Rebecca said. 'I'm going to go and scrub out, now, but I'll pop in to SCBU to see you after my shift.'

'Thank you.' Mrs Kamanya reached out and squeezed her hand. 'You've been so kind.'

'You're very welcome,' Rebecca said.

Later that afternoon, she visited SCBU to discover Mrs Kamanya sitting with the baby doing kangaroo care.

'Well, Miss Kayleigh, you look very settled with your mum,' she said with a smile, stroking the sleeping baby's cheek very lightly, then turned to the Kamanyas. 'How are you both doing?'

'Besotted with my wife and my daughter,' Mr Kamanya answered. 'I'm still a bit scared of holding her, because she's so tiny, but the way I feel about her...' His face was filled with pride.

'Me, too. Mr Jones came in to see us earlier,' Mrs Kamanya said. 'I still can't believe how lovely everyone is.'

'We've got a good team,' Rebecca agreed. 'We all love babies and we want our parents to have the best possible experience. And we're all here to help if you've got any questions, however small or silly they might seem. We'd all much rather you asked than held back and were worried about something.'

'That's good to know,' Mr Kamanya said.

'I'll pop back in tomorrow. But it's good to see her doing so well,' Rebecca said.

'That's what Mr Jones said,' Mrs Kamanya remarked.

Rebecca was beginning to think that she and Nathaniel were very much on the same page. So could this thing between them actually work— or was she hoping for too much?

CHAPTER SIX

NATHANIEL WAS ALREADY with a mum in the labour suite when Rebecca got into work, the next day; she had clinic in the morning, then visited Mrs Kamanya in the SCBU during her lunch break.

'How's it going?' she asked.

'Kayleigh's getting stronger, hour by hour,' Mrs Kamanya said. 'She's not quite able to latch on, yet, but I'm expressing milk for her.'

'That's good. And she'll get there when it comes to latching on,' Rebecca reassured her.

'Mr Jones popped in to see us this morning, too,' Mrs Kamanya said. 'Before his shift. He brought me a croissant—we'd been talking about them the other day, and he said pain au chocolat is the best breakfast, but I voted for croissants. I didn't expect him to do something so lovely.' She smiled. 'He's such a sweetie, isn't he?'

'Yes,' Rebecca said. She was beginning to realise that Nathaniel was a man who paid attention to the little things that mattered to people, and acted on them. He was the reliable type.

Not like Lucas, a little voice whispered in her head, and she silenced it. She'd dated Nathaniel once. There was a long, long way to go before she could consider anything major.

She eventually caught up with him mid-afternoon.

'Guess what? I delivered a baby boy, this afternoon. And Nathaniel's going to be his middle name. Reee-sult!' He grinned and gave her a high-five.

'On a post-delivery high, are we?' she teased, to take her mind off the fact that the way his eyes crinkled at the corners made her knees go weak.

'Absolutely.' His gaze held hers. 'So come and celebrate with me?'

'Sorry. I have ward rounds,' she said. Though she didn't want him to think she was pushing him away. 'Maybe some other time?'

'How about,' he said, 'I cook for you?'

'Would this be your famous run-down fish stew?' she asked, remembering what he'd said on their date.

'Rita's run-down fish stew,' he corrected. 'Yes.'

A second date. Except this one would be

much more intimate. Nathaniel was offering to let her into his space. Could she be brave enough to say yes, and let him closer to her?

She thought about it. Part of her was wary; she'd worked out that he'd been hurt and he'd said he hadn't been in a serous relationship for a while. Did that mean he wouldn't be able to commit if things started to get serious between them? She didn't want to take a risk on her heart—or Jasmine's. She needed someone who was stable, strong and committed.

But another, more insistent part of her wanted to get to know him better. How else could she find out whether he was someone who'd stick around when things started to get tough or someone who'd vanish at the first hint of things not being perfect?

Saying yes would mean pushing the boundaries a bit—for both of them. 'OK. Thank you. I'd like that.'

'Tonight?' he suggested.

'I can't do tonight, but maybe tomorrow night, if I can get a babysitter,' she said. 'Is it OK to let you know later?'

'Sure.'

At the end of her shift, Rebecca collected Jasmine from her parents.

'Mummy! I drawed you a picture today,' Jasmine said. 'It's a dinosaur.'

A pink diplodocus, with what looked like a glittery silver bow round its long neck. Rebecca smiled. 'It's beautiful, darling. Look how well you've drawn his neck. We'll put that up on the fridge as soon as we get home.'

Jasmine beamed and hugged her.

'Can you go and put all your things in your bag and say goodbye to Grampy, while I have a quick catch-up with Nanna?' Rebecca asked.

Jasmine nodded and scampered off.

'Mum, I know it's a massive cheek, but if you're free could I ask you to babysit for me tomorrow night?'

'Babysit? Of course I can.' Caroline looked pleased. 'Is this a date?'

Rebecca squirmed. 'Yes, but it's really early days.'

'I'm glad you're finally moving on. Lucas wouldn't have wanted you to be alone—just as, if you were the one who'd had the accident, you wouldn't have wanted him to spend the next fifty years mourning you.'

'I know,' Rebecca said softly. 'But we're just taking it one step at a time.'

'I just want to see you happy again, love,' Caroline said gently.

'I *am* happy, Mum. I've got the best family in the world, my friends are great, and I love my job.'

'I know, love. But you also need time to be *yourself*,' Caroline counselled. 'You're still young. And you know your dad and I will baby-sit any time you need us to. So will Saskia.'

'I love you, Mum,' Rebecca said, hugging her.

'Love you, too. Let me know what time you need us tomorrow.'

'I will,' Rebecca promised.

Jasmine chattered all the way back to their own house, and helped Rebecca make the gnocchi with mozzarella and tomato sauce, rolling the balls of dough down a fork and giggling. Moments like these were so precious, Rebecca thought, making memories that could help her daughter through any tough times in the future. She hoped that Jasmine would always associate the scent of basil with a sunny late afternoon in their kitchen.

Once they'd eaten, and done the bath and bedtime routine, Rebecca read a last extra story and hugged her daughter. 'Time for sleep, now,' she said gently. 'Sweet dreams. Love you to the moon and back.'

'Love you to the moon and back twice,' Jasmine said.

Rebecca curled up in a chair with her phone and texted Nathaniel.

Babysitting organised. Let me know your ad-
dress and what time.

He replied with the details almost straight
away.

Seven o'clock was just about perfect; it meant
she could make lasagne for her parents and Jasmine tomorrow afternoon.

OK. I'll be there. Should I bring red or white
wine?

No need. Just yourself.

She called him. 'I can't just bring myself.
You're cooking for me. It feels rude not to bring
something.'

'It's fine,' Nathaniel said.

'No, it's not,' she said. 'If you don't tell me,
I'll bring a bottle of red and a bottle of white.'

'It's a spicy stew, so wine doesn't really go
with it. Really. Just bring yourself,' he said
again.

'OK. I'm not going to fight with you,' she
said. But she also didn't intend to turn up
empty-handed. If he didn't want her to bring
wine, she'd bring something else. 'See you tomorrow.'

Rebecca had a half-day on Friday, so she

was able to pick up Jasmine from nursery at lunchtime and take her to the park. The weather was perfect, sunny and bright but without being too hot. She thoroughly enjoyed pushing Jasmine on the swings, helping her on the climbing frame—Jasmine's favourite thing—and watching her come down the slide, then walking through the rose garden on the way home.

They took a detour to the high street, where they bought strawberries and salted caramel ice cream for pudding, and Rebecca bought some things to take to Nathaniel. Back at their house, Jasmine gave her teddies a tea party in the kitchen while Rebecca made lasagne.

'Everything's prepped, Mum,' Rebecca said when her parents arrived. 'Lasagne's in the oven, salad and strawberries are in the fridge, and Dad's favourite ice cream is in the freezer.'

'Wonderful. Thank you. Now, off you go and have a good time,' Caroline said.

'You look so pretty, Mummy. Just like a princess—no, like a queen,' Jasmine said.

'Thank you. I'm going to have dinner with one of my colleagues from the hospital,' Rebecca said. It wasn't a lie—just not the whole truth. 'Be good for Nanna and Grampy.'

'Don't rush back,' Caroline said. 'Your father will fall asleep in front of the TV, and I brought my crochet with me.'

'See you later, Mum.' Rebecca kissed them all goodbye, then headed for Nathaniel's flat. It was a nice evening, and he was only a twenty-minute walk away. The flat was in a purpose-built development; seeing the small square of grass and nondescript shrubs at the front reminded her what he'd said about envying her having a garden of her own.

She took a deep breath and rang the bell for his flat.

The intercom crackled. 'Hey, Rebecca. I'm on the second floor. I'll buzz you in.'

When he hung up, she heard a buzz and then the front door opened. She closed it behind her and climbed the two flights of stairs; as she reached the landing, she saw him standing in one of the doorways.

'Welcome,' he said, and ushered her inside.

The door to her left was closed; she guessed it was his bedroom. 'The bathroom's just here, if you need it,' he said, gesturing to the second door, and then shepherded her into the living room. There was a small kitchen at one end, with a bistro-style table and two chairs set next to a large window; the main living room area was just big enough for a sofa and a TV. There were no books in evidence, and she guessed that his music and films were all streamed digitally.

Everywhere was scrupulously tidy.

'You said not to bring wine, so I brought you these,' she said, and handed him a brown paper carrier bag.

'You didn't have to, but thank you,' he said, looking inside. 'Oh, wow. Posh chocolates. I love these. Thank you. And basil.'

'You said you had enough space for herbs on your windowsill, and I know you're a foodie,' she said.

'And you can't beat fresh basil for pesto, pasta sauce or ratatouille—thank you.' His smile broadened as he took the final thing out of the bag: a pink corduroy mouse. 'I assume this is for my flatmate?'

'Of course.' She smiled. 'It's filled with catnip. I've never had a cat, so I have no idea whether he'll like it or not.'

'Oh, he will,' Nathaniel assured her. 'Come and meet him.'

Leo had draped himself across the back of the sofa.

'Leo, come and make friends. This is Rebecca and she's the reason why you've got fish for dinner tonight,' Nathaniel said to the cat.

Leo purred and allowed Rebecca to stroke him; she was surprised by how soft his fur was.

And the cat seemed thrilled with the toy mouse when Nathaniel gave it to him; Leo immediately started throwing it about and pouncing on it.

'Something smells lovely,' she said.

'I hope it tastes all right,' he said.

'Is there anything I can do to help?'

'Thanks for the offer, but it's all sorted.' He glanced at his watch. 'It should be ready in about ten minutes. If you'd like to take a seat, I'll get you a drink.' He gestured to the neatly set bistro table. 'Would you prefer coffee, beer, or something soft?'

'If you've got any sparkling water, that'd be lovely, thanks,' she said.

'I have,' he said, and took a bottle from the fridge. He poured the contents into two glasses. 'Ice? Lime?'

'Both, please.'

He added the lime and ice to the sparkling water, then handed a glass to her. 'Cheers,' he said, and clinked his glass against hers.

He put the chocolates on the worktop, the pot of basil on his windowsill, and smiled at her. 'OK. I'm afraid I have to be boring now and do things.'

'Are you sure I can't help?' she asked.

'I'm sure. Just chat to me,' he said, and took a bowl out of the fridge. 'The dumplings—I made them earlier,' he explained.

'So you're going to boil them?' she asked,

noting the large pan of water coming to a simmer on the hob.

'I'm going to fry them,' he said, 'which probably sounds as if it'd clog your arteries, but actually they're very light and fluffy—at least, they are when Rita makes them. It's a while since I've made them.' He took a skillet out of a cupboard, added oil and set it to heat. While the dumplings were cooking, he added dark green leaves to the water. 'Cavolo Nero,' he said. 'You need something strong to stand up to the spices. I hope you like it.'

'I like all vegetables,' she said, 'with the exception of really large Brussels sprouts.' She grimaced. 'Or even the small ones, if they've been cooked to a mush.'

'Sprouts are only edible, in my view, if you shred them and stir-fry them with ginger, chilli and garlic,' he said. 'Mushy veg...' He spread his hands. 'Not in my kitchen.'

'I see you have a few drawings on the outside of your fridge,' she said.

He smiled. 'Feel free to have a look, if you want to. I imagine you get the same kind of thing brought home from nursery.'

'Your goddaughter drew them?' she asked.

'Yes. Every month she gives me a picture she did especially for me, with varying amounts of glitter. She's hugely into dinosaurs at the moment.'

'So's Jas. Whenever I ask her what she wants to do at the weekend, if it's raining she always wants to go and see the dinosaurs in the Natural History Museum,' Rebecca said, smiling.

'Sounds like fun,' he said, smiling back. 'Grab a seat, because I'm serving up.' He flicked into something on his phone, and music started playing from a speaker on the windowsill. 'I hope you'll like this—Dad's a part-time musician, and this is the kind of stuff he used to play all the time when I was a kid.'

Indie music from the nineties, the sort of thing her own father played. 'I used to hear a lot of this in the car, too,' she said. 'It brings back lovely memories.'

'I'm glad.' He brought two plates over to the table.

'Cheers.' She lifted her glass in a toast. 'Thank you for inviting me.'

'Thank you for coming.'

She took a mouthful of the stew. 'Wow. This is amazing.'

He looked pleased. 'Glad you like it.'

They chatted easily through dinner, and Rebecca learned that Nathaniel had never set foot in a gym but had played rugby at county level before the accident. 'Obviously contact sports for me are spectator-only, nowadays.' He shrugged. 'But I'm lucky. I'm not going to moan about missing sport. Not after months of wondering if I'd ever be able to even walk again. I can still kick a ball round a park with my goddaughter. I'm luckier than a lot of people.'

She liked the fact he focused on the positives.

'What about you? You do gymnastics? Roller skating? Champion swimmer?'

She laughed, enjoying the twinkle in his eye and the absurdity. 'No. Saskia and I did ballet when we were kids, and I did aerobics classes before I had Jas. I don't really get time for any of that sort of thing, now.' She smiled. 'But that's fine. I get to have fun with her in the park, going for a walk and seeing what we can find, and pushing her on the swings.'

'Sounds good,' he said, and for a moment there was wistfulness in his eyes.

And she could imagine him pushing a child on a swing or walking with a toddler and pointing out butterflies and bees and flowers. It made her heart feel as if it had been squeezed. Did he want more from life than she'd be able to give him?

Nathaniel wouldn't let her clear the table, but brought over a bowl of summer berries and a tub of very posh salted caramel ice cream. 'I know it's a bit of a lazy pudding, but I remember you said it was your favourite.'

Again, she noticed, he paid attention and remembered the little things. Lucas would've remembered her dream holiday destination or her dream car, but even after they'd been married for a year he'd still put sugar in her coffee despite the fact she'd never taken it. 'It's my dad's, too. Actually, that's what he, Mum and Jas are having for pudding tonight.'

'Great minds think alike, then,' he said lightly.

He did at least allow her to help with the washing up, before making them both coffee and leading her into the living room. Although there wasn't a fire, there were some shelves opposite the sofa, and the middle one contained framed photographs.

'Can I be nosey?' she asked.

'Sure.'

She walked over to the shelves. There was a photograph of Charlotte and Robyn's wedding, with Nathaniel looking handsome in top hat and tails; there was a second photograph of him in top hat and tails with a man of similar age, clearly at another wedding, but she couldn't see a family resemblance between them.

'My best friend, Jason,' he said, 'at his wedding to Denise.'

There was photograph of Nathaniel wearing a gown and mortar board at his graduation, with his parents; and another of him holding a baby in a very pretty white dress. 'Is that Sienna?' she asked.

'Yes.' He smiled. 'I can't wait to be an uncle. It'll mean I get double the drawings on my fridge.'

There was another of Sienna as a toddler, with Leo sitting on her lap. 'That's cute.'

'Yeah. She loves Leo—and he adores her. Whenever Jason brings her over, he always sits with her.'

The final photograph was a picture of an older couple at sunset, smiling broadly, with a city spreading out behind them. She recognised them from his graduation photograph. 'Your mum and dad?' she asked.

'Yes. Suzanne and Mark,' he said. 'It was their ruby wedding, last year. Charlotte and I sent them to Paris for the weekend—that's where they went on their honeymoon.' He smiled. 'They had a fine time pretending they were twenty-one again, wandering around in Montmartre and the like. We bought them tickets for the Eiffel Tower at sunset—and apparently there's this *guinguette* by the Seine, a kind of open-air bar which serves food and people can dance as well. So they went dancing, had something to eat, did the Eiffel Tower, got someone to take a photograph and sent it to Charlotte and me, then went back dancing until midnight.'

'That sounds like the sort of thing my mum and dad would do,' she said, smiling.

Clearly Nathaniel was really close to his family. She liked that; Lucas hadn't been that close to his parents, and it was only when he'd got married to her and she'd made the effort to stay in touch with them that his family had become closer. He'd always been a bit bored by family gatherings, unless they were barbecues when he was in charge of the grill; and she'd ended up going to see her own family alone, most of the time, fibbing to them that Lucas couldn't get the time off work to join her while knowing that he was off somewhere getting his adrenalin fix. And she'd always quietly envied her friends with partners who were happy to do the domestic stuff and were close to their families. Sure, they wouldn't have the excitement of being whisked away to Rome or New York for the weekend; but they had something much more important. A solid foundation to their marriage.

'Come and sit down,' Nathaniel said, and drew her back to the sofa.

Leo stretched out along the arm of the seat

next to him, and Nathaniel slid his arm round Rebecca's shoulders. She leaned in closer, and then somehow his mouth was brushing against hers, sensitising the skin and making her want more.

Kissing Nathaniel held just the same excitement as kissing Lucas once had, except there was something underpinning it. Something safe. Something cosseting. Something that made her feel special and treasured, made her feel as if she was wanted for *herself* rather than just the thrill of the chase.

When he broke the kiss, she opened her eyes. His pupils were huge, making his dark eyes seem almost black, and he laid one hand against her cheek.

'I'm calling a halt,' he said.

'It's over?' The words were out before she could stop them, and she was furious with herself for sounding needy.

'Oh, honey. I didn't mean *that*.' He stole another kiss. 'I mean, I'm calling a halt to the kissing, because I don't want this to be rushed.'

'Oh.' That put a very different complexion on things.

'No pressure,' he said, 'but I like you—a lot—and I'd like to keep seeing you.'

'But you said you didn't really do serious relationships.' She frowned, confused.

* * *

Oh, his stupid mouth. Nathaniel groaned inwardly. Well, he was going to have to tell her now. At least some of it. Because she'd practically asked.

'I used to be engaged. She called it off.'

'I'm sorry,' Rebecca said. 'That must have hurt you a lot.'

He could see she was trying really hard not to ask any more, and he appreciated that. On the other hand, he didn't want her leaping to conclusions, thinking that either he or Angie had cheated.

If he told her the truth, he didn't want her pitying him. 'No pity, right?' he asked.

Her expression was full of sympathy rather than pity. 'I promise. I've been "poor Rebecca", and I hated it. I won't do that to you.'

He hadn't considered that, but it gave him the confidence to tell her. 'Angie and I—I thought she was the one. But she signed up to marry a building site manager.'

'She didn't like your career change?'

He winced. 'We didn't get that far.'

Her blue eyes widened as she clearly worked it out for herself. 'She broke it off after the accident?'

He looked away. 'We didn't know if I'd be able to walk again.'

'Hang on. She dumped you before you found out whether you would actually recover from the accident? That's *heartless*.' She sounded furious on his behalf.

'It was honest. If I hadn't recovered and we'd gone ahead with the wedding, then she would've felt trapped and we would have both been miserable.'

She rolled her eyes. 'You're a lot more reasonable than I would've been, in your shoes.'

'There isn't much point in being anything else.' He shrugged. 'Yes, I was hurt and angry at the time, and I resented her for dumping me while I was still in hospital—but, when I think about it, maybe that was better than facing up to a lifetime with someone who didn't want to be with me.'

She flinched, and he frowned. 'Rebecca?'

'I…' She blew out a breath. 'You've been honest with me. I should be honest with you, too. My marriage wasn't great. Lucas felt the same way as your Angie did—trapped.'

He stared at her, shocked. 'I'm sorry. I didn't mean to bring bad memories back for you.'

She shook her head. 'It's not your fault. I don't broadcast the fact that I wasn't enough for my husband.'

Exactly how he'd felt, after Angie left. That

his judgement was off—that he'd been too stupid to realise that he wasn't enough for her.

He wrapped his arms round Rebecca. 'So we're kind of the same, but different.'

Her laugh was rueful. 'Yeah. Jasmine wasn't planned, but I was thrilled when I found out that I was pregnant.'

And Lucas wasn't?

He realised he'd spoken aloud when Rebecca said, 'He said he was pleased. But, as I got more and more round, he felt more and more trapped. Broken nights and the demands of a small baby, bogging you down in domesticity when you want to be out there doing extreme sports and getting your adrenalin fix...' She wrinkled her nose. 'It didn't help.'

'It's hard on all of you,' he said, 'when you want different things.'

'I don't want to make that mistake again,' she said.

'Completely understandable. I don't want to make another mistake, either.'

He paused. 'Except something about you makes me want to keep dating you.'

She looked at him. 'I kind of want that, too.'

'But?' She hadn't said the word, but it was written all over her face.

'I'm not ready to introduce you to Jasmine as anyone other than my colleague.'

'I understand that completely,' he said.

'And there's the risk of gossip at work.'

'Which usually lasts about a week and then everyone starts talking about something else,' he pointed out. 'But we can keep this just between us, if that makes you more comfortable.'

'It does at the moment,' she said.

'OK. We have all the time in the world. No need to rush.'

How very different from Lucas and the way he'd swept her off her feet.

With Lucas, she'd always felt as if she were walking on a tightrope with nothing to break her fall. With Nathaniel, her pulse still raced when he kissed her and her heart felt as if she were doing acrobatics, but there was a safety net—Nathaniel himself. He made her feel giddy as a schoolgirl, but at the same time he made her feel grounded and safe, in a way that Lucas never had. As if she had someone on her side, someone who'd be there in a crisis to support her and help her—and not just assume that she'd be happy to take the full burden of sorting everything out.

'I'd like that,' she said. 'So what do we do now?'

'Given that your ex liked doing risky stuff,

I'm assuming you're not that keen on surprises?' he said.

'No.' She appreciated the fact he'd worked that out for himself. 'I like to know what I'm dealing with.'

'How about a half-surprise?' he suggested. 'Monday night, I'd like to take you out. It's something I think you'll like. If I can get tickets tomorrow, then you'll need a coat and someone to babysit until about eleven p.m. If I can't, then I'll have a rethink and come up with some alternatives and run them by you.'

'All right. That'd be lovely.'

'Good.' He stole a last kiss. 'It's raining, so I'll drive you home. Or I can call you a taxi, if you'd rather.'

She glanced over to the kitchen window and realised there were raindrops spattered against the glass. 'Since you put it so nicely, thank you. A lift would be nice.'

He kept the conversation light all the way to her house. 'See you at work on Monday.' He kissed her lingeringly, and even though it was still raining his kiss made her feel as if it were the middle of the day, with the sun shining brightly. How was it that he could make her feel that kind of warmth, that kind of brightness?

'Monday,' she said, and kissed him one last time before climbing out of the car. She turned to wave at him just before she opened her front door, and he blew her a kiss.

Cute.

Nathaniel Jones was seriously cute.

And she was going to have to be careful, or she'd be in danger of losing her heart to him completely.

CHAPTER SEVEN

REBECCA DIDN'T REALLY have time to think about Nathaniel on Saturday—Jasmine had a swimming lesson and then a play date with her best friend from nursery, giving Rebecca a chance to blitz the house and catch up with laundry. But she did check that Saskia could babysit on Monday, and texted him to let him know that babysitting was fine.

Sunday morning was spent making Eton Mess and brownies, and then they headed off to her parents' house.

But when she checked her phone on Sunday evening, there was a message from Nathaniel.

Got the tickets I wanted. Will pick you up at eight. Bring a coat and wear something warm. I'll bring chairs and blankets. xx

She had absolutely no idea what he had in mind; clearly he wanted to keep it a surprise.

But he had at least told her information she needed to know.

Thank you. Am intrigued.

She wrinkled her nose, then added,

Where are we going? Xx

Out. xx

That was the reply, followed by a smiley face.
OK. She'd stop asking and let him enjoy making the surprise.

See you tomorrow. xx

Rebecca was in Theatre the next day when he was on a break, and he was in a delivery suite during her break, so she didn't get to see him until he picked her up at eight.

When he rang her doorbell, Saskia beat her to answering the door.

'Hey. Nice to meet you properly, Nathaniel. I'm Saskia,' she said.

'Nice to meet you, too,' he said, shaking her hand.

'Enjoy your evening.' She glanced at the bags

slung over his shoulder. 'Are you taking my big sister on some kind of picnic?'

'Oh, no,' Rebecca said, 'because I've already had dinner and you didn't warn me not to.'

'It's not a picnic. Wait and see,' he said.

She rolled her eyes. 'Man of mystery, are we?'

He glanced down at his jeans and light sweater. 'I really should've dressed all in black and worn dark glasses.'

Saskia laughed. 'He's not going to tell us what you're doing tonight, Bec. Have fun, you two. I have a date with a good film and a mug of hot chocolate.'

Rebecca still didn't have a clue what they were doing until they reached the park and she saw the signs. 'We're going to a pop-up cinema showing of *Dirty Dancing*?'

'Is that OK?' he asked.

'I love that film. Especially that bit where Patrick Swayze rescues Baby from her parents.' She smiled. 'Great choice. Thank you.'

'Good. We have fold-up picnic chairs—borrowed from my sister—a fleecy blanket, and I was planning to get us hot chocolate.'

'Let me get them,' she said.

He shook his head. 'My idea, so I'm paying. But you can message your sister to tell her you're doing the same thing—except outdoors.'

Now she realised why he'd told her to wear
something warm and bring a coat. While he
was getting hot chocolate for them, she texted
Saskia.

Pop-up cinema. Dirty Dancing! Xx

The reply came immediately.

Good choice. Keeper! Xx

'OK?' he asked when he came back.
'Very. Thank you,' she said.
There was something incredibly sweet and
romantic about sitting in a picnic chair next to
his, with a fleecy blanket tucked round them,
holding his hand under the blanket and holding
a cup of hot chocolate in her free hand, watching the sky darken as the film started and a few
faint stars begin to appear above them. No pressure: just warmth and a sweetness that made
her heart feel as if it had done a somersault.
She'd seen the film a few times with her
mum and her sister, but she still enjoyed it: everything from the music to the dancing. Nathaniel wrapped one arm round her shoulders
during the second half, when the air was beginning to get chilly, and she leaned her head

against his shoulder, feeling warm and cherished. This really was the perfect evening.

The final scenes of the film came onto the screen, and the whole of the audience chorused the iconic line before watching Johnny and Baby's show-stopping dance, ending with that triumphant lift. And it felt so right, so natural, to turn to Nathaniel when Baby and Johnny were still in the centre of the dancing crowd, leaning into each other for a kiss in exactly the same way as the couple on the screen.

Her eyes closed as Nathaniel's mouth touched hers in the lightest, sweetest, gentlest kiss. And then, as the kiss deepened, it felt as if fireworks were going off inside her head. Huge starbursts, bright and sparkling, the sort that lit up the whole sky in silver, white and gold.

Shaking, she broke the kiss. 'Nathaniel,' she whispered.

He looked as dazed as she felt. 'I... You...'

There were no words.

So she just laid her palm against his cheek and kissed him again, until she was dizzy with need and desire.

And then she realised that everyone around them was standing up, packing up their chairs and their blankets.

Her face heated. 'Sorry.'

'I'm not. I like it when you kiss me.' He

kissed the tip of her nose. 'But we'd better go. Your sister's expecting us back. And everyone else around us...' He gestured to the people streaming past them.

Between them, they packed the fold-up chairs back into their carry-cases and put the blanket back in the tote bag. He slung all the handles over his shoulder, then took her hand. 'I'll walk you home.'

It turned out to be quite a slow walk home, punctuated by a kiss under every fourth lamp-post, but finally they reached her front door.

'Goodnight,' he said. 'And thank you for coming to the film with me.'

'I loved it,' she said honestly. 'Thank you for making it a *nice* surprise.'

'So you'd trust me if I wanted to surprise you in future?'

She didn't even have to think about it. She already knew. Nathaniel was a man who thought about things, who noticed little details and paid attention instead of muddling through. She trusted him. 'Yes.'

He kissed her again. 'Good. I'll see you at work tomorrow.'

'And maybe we can synchronise our off-duty,' she said. 'I'm on a late on Friday.'

'So am I.'

'Maybe,' she said, 'we can have breakfast together.'

'Do you have somewhere in mind?'

She nodded. 'It's a bit of a trek, but we can get a bus and the Tube.'

'It sounds like somewhere you've been before?'

'I haven't, actually, but I've planned to take Jas there for a while. I thought maybe we could scope it out together.'

He smiled. 'I'd like that.'

'I'll sort out the details and tell you tomorrow,' she said.

He kissed her one last time. 'Goodnight.'

'Goodnight,' she said, and quietly let herself into the house.

The next morning, Rebecca got up early to make the batter for pancakes, chop fruit and lay the table for breakfast; by the time she came downstairs again after helping Jasmine get ready for nursery, Saskia was in the kitchen and had made coffee.

'Here you, go, Big Sis,' Saskia said, handing Rebecca a mug of coffee just the way she liked it.

'Angel. Thank you.' Rebecca heated oil in the pan and busied herself cooking pancakes while Jasmine poured a glass of milk with Saskia's help.

'Where did you go last night, Mummy?' Jasmine asked.

'I went to the pop-up cinema with a friend from work.'

Jasmine looked confused, 'What's a pop-up cinema?'

'It's a cinema outside in the park,' Rebecca explained.

'That sounds so cool. Can I go with you next time? Please?' Jasmine added swiftly.

'It'd be a bit too late for you, darling. You'd be asleep before the film had started.' At the disappointed look on Jasmine's face, she said, 'But I read there's going to be a floating pop-up cinema in the summer, showing films every morning. Maybe we can do that.'

'If it's *The Little Mermaid*, I'm so coming with you,' Saskia said. She broke into a chorus of 'Part of Your World', and Jasmine joined in.

'We'll make it a girly day,' Rebecca promised, 'and take Nanna with us.'

'Can we have popcorn?' Jasmine asked, spooning fruit onto her pancakes.

'Absolutely. Or we can make a special picnic,' Rebecca said.

'Did you have popcorn last night?' Jasmine asked.

'No. But we did have hot chocolate. Now, finish your pancakes and go and clean your teeth,' Rebecca directed.

'I'm glad you had a good time last night,' Saskia said when Jasmine had gone upstairs to clean her teeth.

'I did—and thank *you* for making it possible.'

'So are you seeing him again?'

Rebecca nodded. 'Though we're taking it slowly. I don't want to make the same mistake I did with Lucas.'

'Sensible,' Saskia agreed.

Between them, they cleared up in the kitchen; then Rebecca hugged her sister goodbye at the front door, took Jasmine to nursery and headed to work.

The day was incredibly busy, with ward rounds and two full clinics, so she didn't get to see Nathaniel, even briefly. Though she called him later that evening, after Jasmine had gone to sleep.

'Hey. Had a good day?' he asked.

'I did. I thought you'd like to know, Mrs Ridley was in my clinic today,' she said. 'The baby's still head-down, so hopefully she'll get the birth she wants.'

'As much as a baby will let its mum plan a

birth,' he said, and she could practically hear the smile in his voice.

'How was your day?' she asked.

'Clinic, and a mum who got to five centimetres dilated at the end of my shift—so I'll miss out on the birth,' he said.

'But you can still get your baby cuddle if she's on the ward tomorrow,' she said. 'About breakfast on Friday—I need to take Jasmine to nursery, first. Can I meet you at nine at the bus stop outside the park?'

'That sounds good,' he said. 'Is there anything I need to know beforehand?'

'Only that it's my idea so it's my bill—and you can't argue, after yesterday evening.'

'All right. I'll see you tomorrow,' he said. 'Sweet dreams.'

And she had the feeling they might be of him. 'Sweet dreams,' she echoed.

On Friday morning, Nathaniel was at the bus stop at ten to nine. Although he tried to appear as if he was casually browsing the internet on his phone, he felt keyed-up. Nervous. This would be their fourth date—and his relationships hadn't progressed this far in years. And he had the nasty feeling that Rebecca could really matter to him—that she could break his heart.

Maybe he should be sensible and back away now, before either of them got hurt.

Yet something about her drew him. She was warm and sweet and kind. OK, so he'd once thought that about Angela and got it very wrong… But Rebecca wasn't Angela. Just as he wasn't Lucas. And maybe, just maybe, they'd be enough for each other.

While he'd been brooding, she'd somehow managed to walk up the road without him noticing her. She was dressed casually in faded jeans and a stripy T-shirt, and she looked so cute that his heart did a somersault.

'Good morning.' She greeted him with a smile. 'I hope you're hungry.'

'Starving,' he said, smiling back. 'So where are we going?'

'To see some lavender fields,' she said.

He frowned. The ones he knew about were hours away. 'But we're both on duty at half-past one.'

'I know, but we've got plenty of time.'

'You're telling me there are lavender fields in London?' he asked, surprised.

'There are indeed,' she said.

They took the bus to Finsbury Park Tube station, then headed out on the Victoria line.

At the station, she consulted her phone. 'This way,' she said, and it turned out to be a five-minute walk to a park. He still didn't quite see how this was a lavender field, until they turned a corner.

'This is lovely,' he said. 'I had no idea that this was here.'

'I know there are bigger lavender farms outside the city, but I saw an article about this the other day and I thought this'd be a nice place to take Jasmine. She loves butterflies. There's a fabulous butterfly house opening in Notting Hill next year, and we've already been to the ones at the Horniman Museum and London Zoo. I wanted to take her somewhere a bit smaller than Kew but where she'd still see lots of butterflies.'

'This looks perfect. My goddaughter loves butterflies, too.' Should he take the risk? Push their relationship one step further? 'Maybe we can take the girls together, sometime,' he suggested.

'Maybe.'

He could see the wariness in her face. 'What's worrying you about the idea?' he asked, trying to be gentle.

'It's still really early days between us,' she said. 'Sorry, I don't mean to be horrible, but I'm not quite ready for you to meet Jasmine properly, yet.'

'Fair point,' he said. Time to back off. He

didn't want her to be so far out of her comfort zone that she wouldn't see him again. She had more to lose than he did. He really shouldn't be letting himself get involved with someone whose life wasn't as free as his own; yet she drew him.

'Let's go have breakfast before we walk round the lavender,' she said.

'OK.' They headed to the café and found a quiet table. 'So are you going for the full English breakfast?' he asked.

'Not when there's a cranberry, Brie and bacon toasted sandwich with my name on it,' she said. 'How about you?'

'Coffee and a bacon sandwich, with brown sauce, please,' he said.

'Brown sauce?'

'Bacon butty and brown sauce. Builder's best breakfast,' he said with a grin.

To his relief, the slight clowning around seemed to relax her again.

The bread was fresh granary, the bacon was smoked by a local butcher and cooked to the perfect crispness, and the coffee was excellent.

'It doesn't get better than this,' he said. 'Good choice, Dr Hart.'

'You're welcome, Mr Jones.'

He kept the conversation light until they'd finished and headed back out into the park.

Walking through the lavender brought back memories for him. 'The scent of lavender always makes me think of my grandparents,' he said.

'Were you close to them?' she asked.

He nodded. 'They still live in the same little cottage by the sea, and there are these huge pots of lavender by the front door. Mum and Dad have moved near them so they can keep an eye on them, but I remember growing up in London and going to stay with my grandparents in the summer holidays. Charlotte and I would spend hours building sandcastles and collecting shells. Even when I was a moody teen, I liked staying there—I'd take their dog for a long walk on the beach and just let the sea work its magic.' He smiled. 'It's Gran's birthday this weekend, so I'm going down to see them and my parents.'

'You mentioned their dog,' she said. 'I thought you were a cat person?'

'I like both,' he said, 'but with my working hours it's easier to have a cat.'

'Fair point,' she said.

'Grandad was a builder. He used to let me help mix the mortar if he was building a wall for someone locally, and he taught me how to lay bricks.'

'Is that why you became a builder?' she asked.

'A chip off the old block, you mean? Probably.'

'Do you miss building?' she asked.

'Sometimes,' he said, 'but I love what I do now even more than I used to like building. I thought Grandad would be disappointed in me not carrying on in his footsteps, after the accident, but he told me to follow my heart—and he also said that it would be a lot easier on Mum, not having to worry about me every time I went to work, in case I fell off another roof.'

She squeezed his hand. 'I think all parents worry about their children, no matter how old their children are.'

'I guess.' He blew out a breath. 'Funny, I thought by the age of thirty-four I'd be settled with kids. Yet here I am.'

'Did the accident affect your fertility as well as breaking your back?' she asked, her voice very gentle.

'Thankfully that wasn't an issue. The only thing that's held me back is not being able to trust that I've met the right person.'

And now it made him ask himself: was Rebecca the right person?

He felt drawn to her in a way he hadn't felt drawn to anyone since Angela.

But it wasn't going to be easy, because he knew she'd been hurt and she had trust issues, too.

'Do you want children?' she asked.

He might as well be honest about it. 'Yes. I'd like to be a dad, at some point in the future. I love being a godfather and I'm really looking forward to being an uncle, but I want the day-to-day stuff, not just the fun stuff. I want to be there for bedtime and breakfast.'

So now she knew for sure: Nathaniel wanted children.

Would being a stepfather be enough for him, or did he want children of his own? She only had one working fallopian tube, which might cause problems if she tried to conceive in future. But she wasn't ready to tell him about that. Not yet. Instead, she said, 'It isn't all fun, being a parent. There are times when it's really hard, when your child's upset and nothing you can do or say can fix it. Or times when they're angry and throw a hissy fit, and you get judgemental comments from random strangers who either never actually had a close encounter with a toddler tantrum or they've blocked out the memories.'

He smiled. 'I remember Sienna's tantrums. There was one day last summer when Jason and I took her to the funfair on the South Bank. She was overtired and overhyped, and I said no, she couldn't go on the merry-go-round again because she'd already done it three times. She screamed her head off. The *looks* we got. In the end, Jason hauled her over his shoulder and walked away, and I said cheerfully to everyone I passed that my goddaughter got her temper from my best friend and not from me.'

'Jasmine's done that before, too. In the middle of the supermarket,' Rebecca said, 'when I'd said no to sweeties. I ended up apologising to everyone round me and feeling like the worst parent in the world. But one woman was really lovely and helped me put my shopping through the till and got Jas to clap along to a song. She said she still remembered what it was like when hers were that age, and she wanted to tell me that it really did get better—just like someone had once done for her.'

'That's a lovely thing to do,' he said. 'I'm prepared for toddler tantrums and teenage moodiness. I'm close to my parents and my sister, and one day I want to share that closeness with my own children.' He looked at her, his eyes filled with questions. 'What about you? I know, in the circumstances, it couldn't happen—but did you ever want more than one child?'

Yes, she had. But how badly that had gone wrong. She couldn't help flinching.

'Sorry. I didn't mean to be intrusive and upset you,' he said, as if he realised he'd accidentally trodden on a sore spot.

'It's not you. I grew up with a sister, so I always thought that if I ever had children I'd probably have two,' she said.

She didn't want to talk about that lost baby, but she knew she ought to give him some kind of explanation. And he'd shared his broken engagement with her, so she knew he wouldn't pity her if she told him the truth about her marriage.

'As you say, Lucas's accident made that decision for me,' she said. 'But, if I'm honest, things had started to go wrong between us even before I got pregnant. I have to be fair to him: he *did* try. But it wasn't the life he really wanted, and the cracks started showing pretty quickly. If he'd been with us for the toddler tantrum stage, I don't think he would've coped.'

'I'm sorry,' he said.

'So am I,' she said. 'I'm sorry Lucas didn't have the chance to walk away and live the life he really wanted, and I'm sorry I didn't give Jasmine the little brother or sister I know she'd dearly love to have. But at least I have Jasmine, and she makes my world a better place.'

* * *

That was what he wanted, too. A partner and child to complete him. A family to love.

His break-up with Angela had made him think he'd wanted too much. But maybe he hadn't.

Though it was too soon to think about that where Rebecca was concerned. This was only their fourth date. Way, way too soon to think about families and potential extensions.

'Look—butterflies,' he said, as much to distract himself as anything else. And it seemed to work, because she changed the subject.

He kept the conversation light as they walked round the parkland. 'This really is a nice park—lots of grass for the kids to run around on, a playground, pretty flowers and all that lavender.'

'It's the perfect place for a four-year-old girl to spend an afternoon,' she agreed. 'I'm definitely bringing Jas here.'

Even though he'd intended to keep a tiny bit of distance between then, her hand accidentally brushed his as they walked, and he ended up linking his fingers with hers, moving closer until they were properly holding hands.

And he just couldn't shake the image that flickered into his head: Rebecca walking beside him, Jasmine running just in front of them, and the kind of glow in Rebecca's face that came with the end of the first trimester...

On Saturday morning, Nathaniel sent Rebecca a photograph of the lavender outside his grand-parents' front door, plus one of what looked like a massively long, sandy beach. The message said:

You'd love it here.

The nearest she got to the beach right now was the local swimming pool for Jasmine's Saturday morning lesson. She replied.

Looks gorgeous.

And it was weird that she missed him.

She'd known him a month: hardly any time at all. Yet, weirdly, she felt as if she'd known him for years.

No rushing, she warned herself silently. She knew he still had his own issues to work through. The woman he loved had dumped him when he'd needed her most, and he hadn't let anyone close since. He might not let *her* close, either; and it would be stupid to start letting herself want what she might not be able to have.

* * *

The following Monday, Nathaniel had a case which concerned him.

Priya Kapoor was a first-time mum. He'd checked her height, weight, blood pressure and the foetal heart rate, and all was fine. He'd checked the baby's growth and the size of Mrs Kapoor's uterus. The blood test results from her twenty-eight-week test showed that her iron levels were normal.

But he wasn't happy with her urine sample.

'So you're thirty-one weeks, Mrs Kapoor,' he said.

'Yes.'

'There isn't any extra sugar or protein in your urine sample,' he said, 'but it's quite dark. Can I ask, are you finding it hard to keep fluids down?'

'No, and I'm drinking plenty, especially as it's been so warm lately,' she said.

'How have you been feeling?' he asked.

'Absolutely fine,' she said with a smile, but he noticed that she was rubbing the skin on the back of her hands. He couldn't see any sign of a rash, but it worried him.

'How about your hands?' he asked gently.

'My mum says it's hormones,' she said. 'She says all pregnant women get itchy hands.'

'Itching is common in pregnancy,' he agreed.

'And yes, it's down to hormones. Your mum is right about that.'

'She says I need to wear loose cotton clothes, and use unperfumed soap and aqueous cream,' Mrs Kapoor said.

'Again, she's right,' Nathaniel said. 'Oat-based soaps and creams can also help. Tell me, do your feet itch as well?'

She nodded.

'And do you find it's less itchy at particular times of day?'

'Most of the time I can cope with it in the day, but it drives me mad at night,' she admitted.

Just what he'd hoped she wouldn't say. 'Is the itch anywhere else?'

'My hands, my feet and the backs of my legs. And I don't understand why, because there isn't a rash or anything.'

'I'd like to do a blood test today,' he said, 'to check your liver function. There is a condition called intrahepatic cholestasis of pregnancy—ICP for short, or you might hear it called obstetric cholestasis. It causes severe itching, especially on your hands and feet. Usually, bile acid flows from your liver to your gut to help you digest food. If you have ICP, the bile acid doesn't flow properly and builds up in your body,' he explained.

'Is that dangerous for the baby?' she asked.

'I don't want you to worry about this, but ICP is linked to increased risks for the baby,' he said. 'If the blood test shows you do have ICP, we'll need to induce labour at about thirty-seven weeks. And I want to see you twice a week between now and then to check your liver function and monitor the baby.'

She bit her lip. 'Is it something I did wrong?'

'No—and it's quite common. One in about a hundred and forty women get it, though it's twice as common in women of Asian heritage,' he added. 'It does tend to run in families, so it might be worth asking your mum if she was ever diagnosed with it.'

Mrs Kapoor looked worried. 'Can you give me anything to stop it?'

'I'm afraid the only treatment is delivering the baby,' he said. 'Can I ask you a really personal question?'

'OK.'

'Have you noticed that your poo is paler than usual?'

'That's not what I was expecting you to ask,' she said, 'but yes. Is that another symptom?'

'It can be,' he said. 'So we might need to give you a vitamin K supplement to make sure your blood clots properly.'

'Is it—? Will it mean the baby's sick or…
worse?' she asked.

'There is a small risk of stillbirth in the late
stages of pregnancy,' he said, 'but please don't
worry. We'll monitor you and the baby very
closely, and we're here if you're worried about
anything at all. I should have your blood test
results back on Thursday, so I'd like you to
come to see me at clinic—and, depending on
the results, maybe have a chat with one of the
doctors about your options.'

'A blood test.' She swallowed hard. 'I hate
needles.'

'I'll be gentle,' he promised, 'and, before I do
anything else, I want you to tell me all about
the nursery you're planning for the baby.'

By the time she was halfway through, he'd
done the blood test.

'I didn't even feel that!' she said.

Because he'd distracted her. 'Good. Mrs Kapoor, I can't give you a definite diagnosis until
I get your bloods back, but I think it's very
probable that you have ICP. And I know it's a
lot to take in, so I'm going to print off a leaflet for you, plus I'll give you the number of the
local support group—it often helps to talk to
someone who's been through it and understands
how you feel.'

'OK. Thank you.'

'Try not to worry,' he said, 'and we'll see you on Thursday.'

He saw Rebecca towards the end of his shift. 'I know I always seem to grab you for complications,' he said.

She spread her hands. 'Which is how it should be. We're a midwife-led unit and the doctors are here for the stuff that needs medical intervention.'

'I might need to borrow you on Thursday afternoon,' he said. 'I've got a mum who might have ICP. The bloods are due back on Thursday afternoon—if it's what I think it is, I might need you to have a chat with her.'

'It's my admin afternoon, so let me know the time of her appointment and I'll make sure I'm there,' she said.

CHAPTER EIGHT

FOR MOST OF the week, Rebecca and Nathaniel were rostered on different parts of the ward. On Tuesday, he called her in to see one of his mums-to-be when the tocograph reading suggested the baby might be in distress. 'I'm not happy with the baby's heart rate, and the labour's been pretty long. I want a foetal blood sample.'

It was the best way of checking that the baby was getting enough oxygen. 'OK. Have you talked the mum through the procedure and explained that it won't hurt the baby at all, or do you want me to do it?'

'Already there and we have consent,' he said.

'Great.' Once Nathaniel had introduced her to the mum-to-be and helped her to lie on the left side with her right leg supported, Rebecca inserted an amnioscope and draped the perineum to ensure a sterile field. Once the baby's scalp was visible, she cleaned it with sterile water, added a thin layer of petroleum jelly, sprayed local anaesthetic and took a sample. She handed the capillary tube to Nathaniel for testing before taking a second sample, checking that the baby's scalp wasn't bleeding, then helped position the mum more comfortably.

'The oxygen levels are fine,' Nathaniel said.

'That's really good,' Rebecca said. She reviewed the tocograph results and sat down on the edge of the bed, holding the mum's hand. 'I'm happy for you to continue labour as it is, but we'll keep the baby monitored continuously. I'd like to put you on a drip to help with your fluid levels, and keep you lying on your left side for a while—what that does is reduce the pressure of your womb on a major vein in your body, so there's good blood flow to the placenta and your baby.'

The mum looked worried. 'So I don't have to have a section?'

'Not necessarily,' Nathaniel said. 'You're almost fully dilated. I know you want a natural delivery if you can, so we'll see how things go—though we might need to help you with delivery, with a ventouse cap or forceps.'

'If the monitoring or any future blood sample tells us that the baby's really not coping well, or the assisted delivery doesn't work,' Rebecca said, 'then we'll have to do a section. But Nathaniel will support you and work with you to try and get you the birth you want, so hopefully next time you see me it'll be on the postnatal ward and I'll get to have a cuddle with your gorgeous little one.'

The mum looked slightly reassured. 'OK. Thank you.'

'Come and get me if you need me,' Rebecca said to Nathaniel. 'I'll get the anaesthetist on standby, plus someone from the neonatal unit.' If things didn't go according to plan, they'd need to move quickly and move the mum to Theatre.

Half an hour later, Nathaniel rapped on the open office door. 'She's fully dilated, but I'm not happy with the baby's heart rate. Mum's consented to assisted delivery, and she knows it means an episiotomy. We've talked it all through and she'd prefer a ventouse, but she's prepared for forceps if you think it's better, and a section if we have to.'

'OK.' She followed him into the room and examined the mum. 'I'm happy for us to give the ventouse a try,' she said. 'I know Nathaniel's already talked it through with you, but I also remember how tough it can be to take things in during labour, so I'll run you through the procedure again and answer any questions either of you might have.'

While she talked the parents-to-be through the procedure, Nathaniel got everything ready and called the anaesthetist, the neonatal specialist and Tanvir, Rebecca's junior.

'It feels like Piccadilly Circus in here,' the mum said, clearly trying to smile.

'Hopefully we won't need them,' Rebecca reassured her, squeezing her hand, and introduced her to everyone.

'It's belt and braces, that's all. But you've got this,' Nathaniel said.

Rebecca sorted out the pain relief and did an episiotomy before attaching the vacuum cup to the baby's head.

During the next couple of contractions, she used gentle suction to help pull the baby out while the mum pushed.

'That's great. You're doing really well,' Nathaniel encouraged.

And finally, the baby arrived. There was the heart-stopping moment before the first cry, and then the baby started pinking up nicely.

'Gorgeous. Well done,' Rebecca said, moved as always by those first few minutes.

While Nathaniel and the neonatal specialist did the newborn checks, everyone else congratulated the new parents and left to get on with the tasks they'd put aside. Nathaniel handed the baby to the mum for skin-to-skin care;

Rebecca delivered the placenta and then repaired the episiotomy.

'Well done. He's beautiful,' she said, stroking the baby's cheek.

She exchanged a glance with Nathaniel, seeing that he was as moved as she was by the first few precious minutes of life. And how excellent he'd been, she thought, encouraging the mum and judging exactly when intervention was needed. It felt as if she'd worked with him for years instead of just a few weeks. As if she'd known him for ever. And that, she felt, was a good sign for the future.

On Thursday lunchtime, Nathaniel caught up with Rebecca in the staff kitchen. 'You know the mum I discussed with you on Monday? I've had the bloods back from the lab, and we're definitely looking at ICP. I've already ruled out hepatitis, and Epstein-Barr.'

'OK. What time do you need me in?' she asked.

'Half-past three,' he suggested.

She nodded. 'I'll be there.'

When she knocked on the door of the consulting room, that afternoon, Nathaniel it and introduced her to Priya Kapoor and her husband, Devendra.

'Nice to meet you both,' Rebecca said. 'I be-

lieve Mr Jones has already talked to you about
the possibility of ICP, and I'm here to answer
any questions you might have.'

Mrs Kapoor dragged in a breath. 'We looked
it up on the internet. And it said if you have ICP
there's a huge risk of a stillbirth.'

'There is a risk, yes,' Rebecca said gently.
'But it's not as huge as the internet claims. We
intend to monitor you very closely. We'll check
the levels of the liver enzymes and bile acid in
your blood every week, give you a vitamin K
supplement to make sure your blood clotting
works correctly, and at your twice-weekly appointment we'll also monitor the baby's heartbeat, growth and amniotic fluid levels.'

'And that will mean we definitely won't have
a stillbirth?' Mr Kapoor asked.

'Nobody can promise complete prevention of
any risks,' Rebecca said. 'But if I'm the slightest bit concerned with any of your test results,
Mrs Kapoor, we can induce your labour. And
we'll monitor the baby's heart rate continuously
during labour.'

'Is there any medication you can give Priya
to stop the itching?' Mr Kapoor asked.

'Nothing reliable, I'm afraid,' Nathaniel said.
'But once the baby's born the itching will go
very quickly, plus the high levels of bile acid
and enzymes will drop back down to normal.'

'I know it's really worrying for you,' Rebecca said, squeezing Mrs Kapoor's hand briefly. 'And the itching makes it really hard to sleep, so mums find that very debilitating as well. Try to rest whenever you can. If you get to thirty-five weeks and you really feel you've had enough, we can deliver the baby early.'

'Doesn't that mean the baby will have to go in Special Care?' Mrs Kapoor asked.

'Yes, but you can spend as much time as you like with your baby, and you'll have the support of all the unit's staff,' Rebecca reassured her. 'We can take you to have a look round the unit, so it'll be familiar and less scary, if you like.'

'Thank you.'

'And we're here if you're worried about anything. Just talk to us and we'll do our best to reassure you,' Nathaniel said.

'Do you have any questions now?' Rebecca asked.

'No. But it's a lot to take in. To think I'm going to have weeks and weeks of this terrible itching…' Mrs Kapoor grimaced. 'I'm hardly getting any sleep as it is.'

'Cool water, calamine lotion, aqueous cream—try the one with a little bit of menthol—and loose cotton clothing will help,' Rebecca advised.

'Thank you.' Though Mrs Kapoor still

looked downcast. Rebecca could understand why—the prospect of having to put up with that unbearable itching for months. If only she had a magic wand or a drug that would help. 'There aren't any clinical trials I know of,' she said, 'but I'll ask around. And if I hear of anything that might help, I promise I'll call you.'

Days like this, when she couldn't make much of a difference, were really frustrating; but it got better towards the end, when Josette Kamanya popped down to tell her that she was going to be taking Kayleigh home in the morning.

Over the next few days, both Nathaniel and Rebecca were rushed off their feet at the ward and ended up working with completely different mums. But although they barely saw each other at work, they video-called in the evenings after Jasmine was asleep, and they'd taken to messaging each other links to songs they thought each other would like—obscure indie music bands from Nathaniel and singalong pop from Rebecca. It had become a kind of game, trying to follow each other's choices with something appropriate, and Rebecca loved it because it made her feel young at heart again.

On Thursday evening when Nathaniel called,

he said, 'I've got some news for you. Mrs Ridley came into the delivery suite this morning.'

Rebecca remembered the mum who'd had ECV. 'How did she get on?'

'A textbook delivery, which I hope made up for the bumpy pregnancy.'

'That's wonderful. But, come on, you can't tell me a tiny snippet about the delivery and skimp on the details,' she reminded him. 'Tell me all.'

'She weighed just over three and a quarter kilograms, had an Apgar score of ten, her name is Daisy, and they're both doing so well that they went home this afternoon.'

'Brilliant. It's always good to hear news like that.'

'Are you free this weekend?' he asked.

'Apart from Jasmine's swimming lesson on Saturday morning, I could be.'

'Could you have lunch with me on Saturday?' he asked. 'I don't mean just you; I'm inviting Jasmine as well.'

Introducing him to Jasmine would mean taking their relationship to the next stage. And although a part of Rebecca was pleased that Nathaniel wanted to meet her daughter properly, part of her went into panic mode. Was this rushing things? Yes, she worked with him so she'd got to know him pretty well, but she'd still only known him for a little over a month. And, yes, it wasn't like the way Lucas had swept her off her feet and into his bed within a weekend, but that still felt a little too fast.

'I'm not sure,' she said. 'Introducing you to my daughter as my friend from work is one thing, but introducing you as...' She stopped. What? 'Boyfriend' sounded too teenagery. 'Partner' sounded permanent—and that couldn't happen until they were both sure of each other, he'd met Jasmine properly and she was happy that Jasmine liked him.

'What do you have in mind?' she asked.

'Mum and Dad are coming to London to stay with me for the weekend,' he said. 'Charlotte's at the fidgety, fed-up stage of pregnancy, so we're going out for a picnic with her and Robyn. It would be lovely if you and Jasmine could join us.'

Meeting his whole family at once... She knew Nathaniel was close to his family; after the way he'd talked about them, she was pretty sure they'd be as easy to get on with as he was. But meeting his family was tantamount to making their relationship official. She wasn't sure she was ready for that.

'As friends,' he said, as if guessing what was holding her back.

It was tempting.

More than tempting.

But there was a massive hole in his plans. 'If your sister is anywhere near as observant as mine, she'll know we're not just friends.'

'She's not going to grill you. That's the benefit of meeting her at this stage of pregnancy,' he pointed out. 'She's a bit preoccupied.'

Meet his family. Introduce him to Jasmine. Take another step forward—a huge step forward.

'They're honestly not scary. My family's *nice*.' He paused. 'Were Lucas's family scary?'

'No. Actually, I still see his parents. I want to make sure Jasmine grows up knowing her grandparents.'

'Then ignore whatever's worrying you,' he said. 'Take your own advice. Come and have a picnic with us. Eat cake, enjoy the sunshine, and… I dunno, play I Spy with Jasmine?'

'That's one of her favourite games.'

'Let's do it. I promise you'll have a great time. Come with us,' he coaxed.

Ignore the scary stuff and get on with it. Which wasn't like Lucas's thrill-seeking: it was acknowledging there were problems, mainly in her head, and not shying away from them. 'All right,' she agreed. 'Just let me know where and what time. Can I make something for the picnic?'

'That'd be lovely. Mum's planning French bread, cheese, ham and tomatoes, and some nibbly bits.'

'Does anyone have allergies I need to work round?'

'Nope. I'm making chocolate brownies and sorting out the drinks. Is there anything Jasmine particularly likes?'

'Apple juice or water would be great. Thanks.'

'Sounds good.' She loved the fact he was so domesticated. Lucas would've bought something at the very last minute, if he'd remembered at all. Nathaniel was much more reliable. 'I can make some of my mum's cheese biscuits, hummus, and bring crudités and strawberries.'

'Perfect,' he said.

He texted her later that evening to say he'd meet them at half-past eleven at King's Cross.

On Friday night, Rebecca and Jasmine made the dough for the cheese biscuits and baked them on Saturday morning so the biscuits could cool during Jasmine's swimming lesson. While they were baking, Rebecca whizzed together some hummus, chopped celery and carrots into sticks, hulled a couple of large punnets of strawberries, and packed everything in boxes ready to take with them.

And at twenty-five past eleven they were walking down to King's Cross. It was the perfect day for a picnic, with bright sunshine and just the lightest breeze.

Nathaniel was already there; in faded jeans, deck shoes, a T-shirt bearing an old nineties band logo and sunglasses, he looked utterly gorgeous. Rebecca's heart felt as if it had done an anatomically impossible somersault, and it turned into a triple when he smiled and said, 'Hi. Thanks for coming.'

'Hi.' She smiled back. 'Jas, this is Nathaniel, my friend from work who invited us on the picnic. Nathaniel, this is my daughter, Jasmine.'

Nathaniel did a formal bow, then took Jasmine's hand and shook it solemnly. 'I'm delighted to make your acquaintance, Miss Hart. And you have a very pretty name—like the princess in *Aladdin*.'

Jasmine went pink with pleasure. 'I love that film. The genie's so funny!'

'Me, too. Shall we go and meet the others?' Nathaniel said. 'Everyone else is already at the boat.'

'Boat?' Rebecca asked, mystified. He'd told her they were going on a picnic. Given that they'd arranged to meet at King's Cross, she'd expected a walk along the canal, perhaps, or a wander through Camley Street Natural Park.

'Did I forget to tell you the picnic is on a boat? Sorry.'

Just like Lucas. Forgetting the important details.

She pushed her impatience aside. She wasn't being fair. He was probably just as nervous about her meeting his family as she was.

He looked awkward. 'I apologise. I should have asked. Do either of you get seasick?'

'No,' Rebecca said.

'Good,' he said, sounding relieved, and led them down the canal path towards a small modern boat. 'One of the guys I used to work with had got to the stage where his knees were protesting every time he laid a floor, so he decided to switch careers and started a hire-boat business. The engine's electric and the boat itself is made of lots of recycled stuff.'

'That's pretty amazing,' Rebecca said.

'He's one of the good guys—he wants to make a difference. Luckily for me, he had a cancellation this week and I was on his waiting list. And it means we can *really* distract Charlotte. On a boat, she's forced to sit and relax.'

Three women were sitting in the middle of the boat, round a table, and a man wearing a captain's hat was seated at the helm. Rebecca recognised his parents from the photographs in Nathaniel's living room, and his sister and sister-in-law from the abseil.

'Rebecca, Jasmine, this is my mum and dad—Suzanne and Mark—my sister, Charlotte, and my sister-in-law Robyn,' Nathaniel said. 'Everyone, this is my friend Rebecca from work and her daughter, Jasmine.'

'Nice to meet you,' Rebecca said, shaking everyone's hand in turn as they got onto the boat.

'Hello,' Jasmine said shyly, clinging to Rebecca's side.

'Where would you like the picnic food, Nathaniel?' Rebecca asked.

'I've put everything else here in the locker,' Nathaniel said, taking the bag Rebecca offered him and stowing it with the rest of the picnic stuff. 'Jasmine, you need to wear a safety jacket,' Nathaniel said, and deftly helped her to put it on before checking it was secure.

'And your hat,' Rebecca added.

She ended up sitting next to Nathaniel; although he didn't hold her hand, he slid his foot next to hers under the table, the pressure just enough to tell her that he wanted to hold her hand but he would let her set the pace.

'I'm so glad we're doing this,' Charlotte said. 'I'm getting so fed up, staying at home and just waiting for the baby to arrive.'

'I guess if anything happens this afternoon,

at least we have a midwife and an obstetrician on board,' Robyn said.

'Don't talk it up,' Suzanne warned with a smile. 'We don't want even a Braxton-Hicks while we're in the middle of the Regent's Canal!'

Everyone laughed. As the conversation went on, Rebecca felt very much part of the group and accepted by Nathaniel's family; she really liked the closeness and the banter.

The scenery was utterly gorgeous. The banks of the canal were lined with trees, and narrowboats painted in pretty colours were moored at the sides, with pots of pansies and marigolds on their roofs. Some of the narrowboats were clearly cafés; one stretch of the waterside seemed to have a collection of boats offering various different crafts for sale, along with a bookshop and a floating beauty parlour.

'We need to come back here on foot,' Mark said, spotting a narrowboat with a record shop.

'You and your record shops,' Suzanne said, smiling at him.

Nathaniel got Jasmine playing I Spy, and proceeded to cheat horrendously, making her laugh even as she protested. Rebecca warmed to him even more, liking the fact that he had the patience to entertain a little girl.

The thought slid into her mind: what a fabulous father he'd make.

And he'd said he wanted a family…

On the one hand, it gave her confidence that this thing between them might work out—that he could be a father to Jasmine. On the other, it terrified her. What if he wanted more children and she couldn't have any?

She damped down the fear. Not now. They were meant to be having a day out. Family time. Fun.

'Look—we're right on the edge of London Zoo,' he said.

'I like the zoo,' Jasmine announced. 'My favourites are the penguins. I love watching them waddle, and then seeing them swim.'

'I like penguins, too,' Nathaniel said. 'And swans—look, there's a gorgeous one over there. And a duck, with a whole row of ducklings following her.'

Jasmine peered over the side of the boat. 'They're so cute!'

'How many are there?' Nathaniel asked.

And Rebecca watched, fascinated, as Nathaniel drew her daughter out, so the little girl forgot her initial shyness and chattered happily to him.

'I know a song about swans and ducklings,' Mark called from the helm.

'Just be grateful Dad didn't bring his guitar,' Nathaniel said with a grin. 'That's why I let him drive today. He can't drive the boat and play guitar at the same time.'

Did that mean Nathaniel's dad was a terrible musician? Rebecca wondered. Yet Nathaniel had said something about his dad being in a band. But then Mark proceeded to sing 'The Ugly Duckling', and encouraged everyone to join in.

She nudged Nathaniel. 'He's really good,' she said.

'I know. Years back, his band played the university circuit,' Nathaniel explained. 'They still play the local pub once every couple of months, but if you get Dad started on music you're never going to get a conversation about anything else.'

'Warning heeded,' she said. 'Though I don't mind talking music.'

Lunch was idyllic, moored in the shade of a tree; it was exactly the same sort of afternoon Rebecca was used to spending with her own family, full of chatter and laughter and warmth, with everyone sitting round the table in the centre of the boat and passing drinks, plates and platters. She very much liked Nathaniel's sister, who was straightforward and down to earth; Robyn, who was a little shy; Suzanne, who reminded her of her own mother; and Mark, who was full of terrible dad jokes and she could see him getting on very well with her own father.

'I need the recipe for these, Rebecca, please,' Charlotte said after her first cheese star. 'They're the best thing I've ever tasted.'

Rebecca smiled, pleased. 'My mum makes them for every family party—and I think my gran gave her the recipe. They're really easy to make. Jas helped me.'

'They're amazing.' Charlotte took another, then grinned at Robyn. 'As I'm eating for two, I think I should have your share.'

'If it stops you huffing and puffing about waiting for the baby to arrive, you can have mine as well,' Nathaniel teased.

On the way back to King's Cross, Jasmine busied herself with the colouring book and pencils Rebecca had brought with them. Charlotte fell asleep with her head on Robyn's shoulder, Suzanne was taking a turn at the helm under Mark's direction, and Nathaniel whispered in her ear, 'Turn to face me.'

She did, and he stole a quick kiss. When her eyes widened in shock that he'd taken such a risk, he said softly, 'Nobody's paying attention, I guarantee that nobody saw that, and you look seriously cute right now so I couldn't resist.'

He looked seriously cute, too. And Rebecca

manoeuvred her bag to hide the fact she was holding his hand all the way back to King's Cross.

'Thank you for a really lovely day,' she said, when they alighted.

'I had a really nice time. Thank you,' Jasmine said, and gave Nathaniel a hug.

He scooped her up, spun her around so she squealed in delight, and kissed the tip of her nose before setting her back on her feet. 'I had a lovely time, too, Princess Jasmine. It was really nice meeting you. Your mum tells everyone at work about you and that you're really good at baking. And now I know she's right. Those cheese stars were so yummy.'

Jasmine beamed at him, clearly pleased, and she didn't stop talking about her new friends all the way home. Later that night, Rebecca called Nathaniel. 'I really enjoyed today. Your family is utterly lovely.'

'They are.' He paused. 'You and Jasmine fitted in perfectly.'

'I felt as if I'd known everyone for years,' she admitted.

'They liked you, too. And, in case you're worrying, as far as they're concerned, you and I are just good friends.'

No expectations, no demands. He'd shared his family with her.

Maybe she should be brave and offer to let him meet her family, too. 'Perhaps you can come and meet Mum, Dad and Saskia— properly, I mean,' she said. 'We could have a barbecue in my back garden, the next week-end you're off.'

'I'd like that,' he said. 'Let me check my off duty.' There was a pause, while she assumed he was checking dates on his phone. 'I'm working for the next two weekends, but I'm off duty the weekend after.'

'The Sunday, then. If that works for you.'

'It does. I'll put it in my diary now.' He paused. 'But in the meantime I'd like to go somewhere with you. I don't mind where we go or what we do—I just like spending time with you.'

'That's how I feel, too,' she admitted.

'Are you free any evening this week?'

'Friday,' she said.

'I'm on an early, so that's fine for me.'

'It's a date,' she said. 'See you tomorrow. And thank you again for today.'

'My pleasure. See you tomorrow,' he said.

CHAPTER NINE

NATHANIEL HADN'T SAID where they were going on Friday. He'd texted Rebecca on Thursday, saying,

It's dressy. I'll pick you up at eight.

Then he'd added,

Oh, and eat lots of carbs for dinner.

Why? she'd asked in her reply.

Can't tell you without ruining the surprise. Humour me. xx had come the answer.

Going out that late meant that she was able to have dinner with Jasmine and Saskia—pizza, to fulfil Nathaniel's recommendation about carbs—and Saskia did her make-up.

'I can't actually remember the last time you got dressed up like this,' Saskia said.

Rebecca wrinkled her nose. 'Are you sure this isn't too over the top?'

'It's a little black dress, Bec. You can't get more classic than a little black dress, heels and pearls, with your hair up,' Saskia said. 'Very Audrey Hepburn.'

'The last time I wore this dress, I was out with Lucas.'

'Who probably left you in a corner all night while he worked the room,' Saskia said. 'At least Nathaniel won't do that.'

'Considering you've only met him briefly, a couple of times, you seem to know him rather well.'

Saskia grinned. 'Psychologists know everything.' She gave Rebecca a hug. 'And, from the way you've talked about him, he pays attention—which is a good thing.'

Nathaniel rang the doorbell at eight on the dot.

'Go. Have fun,' Saskia directed. 'I have a book I'm dying to finish. Go.'

'You look gorgeous,' Nathaniel said when Rebecca opened the door.

'So do you.' She was used to seeing him in scrubs at work and smart-casual clothes on their dates—but tonight he was wearing a formal suit and tie. The formality emphasised his good looks. 'Where we going?'

'That's still classified,' he teased.

Clearly he could tell she was slightly antsy, because he took her hand, dropped a kiss into her palm and curled her fingers over the kiss. 'We're going out for cocktails, somewhere that will have the perfect view of the sunset over London.'

Which didn't tell her *exactly* where they were going, but it was enough to settle her worries about his surprise.

He held her hand all the way on the Tube, and all the way down the street.

'We're going to the Sky Garden?' she asked when they finally stopped.

'I booked us a table. One with a really good view,' he said.

'This has been on my list of places I wanted to go to for *ages*,' she said. 'Thank you.'

He smiled. 'Pleasure.'

When they walked out of the lift, she could see massive tree ferns and lush vegetation in a huge space filled with light. People were sitting at tables in front of the windows, drinking cocktails, and there was a band playing an acoustic set at one end.

'What would you like to drink?' he asked.

She could stick to something safe—wine, or Pimm's. But today she wanted to push the boundaries. 'I've never really done cocktails. Surprise me,' she said.

'Is there anything you really like or hate?' he asked.

'I'm not really much of a one for whisky,' she said.

'OK. I'll talk to the bar staff and bring back a surprise,' he said.

He came back with a glass topped with a paper umbrella, containing a drink that shaded from deep red to orange, reminding her of a sunset, and a copper-coloured glass that contained what look like ice and lime. 'Your choice,' he said. 'A Moscow Mule or Sex on the Beach.'

'I don't have a clue what's in either.'

'Try both,' he suggested, 'and you can tell me what's in them.'

'Ginger, lime, and...something else,' she said after trying the drink in the copper glass.

'Vodka,' he said.

The other was citrusy, tart and peachy. 'I really like this one,' she said.

'Vodka again—but with peach schnapps, orange and cranberry.'

'I think this could be my new favourite drink,' she said with a smile. 'Thank you.'

How pretty she looked tonight, Nathaniel thought, all lit up and sparkly. And he was pleased to see she was relaxing more with him, enough to dance with him when the light started to dim. They went back to their table to watch the sun setting over the city; the Thames turned into a ribbon of silver in the fading light, and then the city started lighting up beneath them, the top of the Shard brilliant white and St Paul's looking majestic.

They danced again, and Nathaniel enjoyed holding her close. She was warm and soft, and she smelled of vanilla and sun-warmed peaches.

Though he knew her daughter had a swimming lesson on Saturday morning. He wasn't going to be selfish about this. 'Come on, Cinders. I'd better get you home before the Tube turns into a pumpkin,' he teased.

'Yes. Though I really don't want tonight to end,' she said.

He looked at her, and his throat felt as if it were filled with sand.

Was she saying…?

'I don't want it to end yet, either,' he said. 'One more dance.'

'One more dance,' she agreed.

Except one more dance wasn't enough. He wanted her. Really wanted her.

'Rebecca,' he whispered. 'You could come back to my place for a nightcap.'

She pulled back slightly. 'A nightcap.' Her blue eyes were unreadable.

'Or I can see you home. No pressure.' He'd give her the choice.

'A nightcap sounds good,' she said.

And the world sparkled and spun with promise.

He held her hand all the way back to his flat. Leo gave a lazy miaow when they came in, but stayed in his basket.

'Nightcap.' He didn't actually drink that much. He rummaged in his fridge. 'Um. There's a bottle of champagne…'

She put her hand over his. 'I'm guessing you bought that to celebrate when your niece arrives.'

'I can replace it.'

'I don't want a drink,' she said. 'I want you to dance with me again.'

He connected his phone to a speaker and streamed some slow dance music.

And this time, when she moved that little bit closer, they were alone instead of being on a dance floor in a posh bar. This time, there was nothing to stop him kissing her. Nothing to stop him brushing his lips against hers, tasting and teasing until she opened her mouth to let him deepen the kiss. It made him dizzy, so he held her tighter, almost drowning in the sweetness of that kiss.

* * *

When Nathaniel broke the kiss and pulled back slightly to look at her, his pupils were huge.

'Rebecca,' he whispered. 'Right now, I really want you.'

She knew what he was asking. Part of her was scared; it had been years since she'd made love, and even longer since she'd made love with anyone except Lucas.

But she wanted this, too. It had been building up for ages: every time they went out together and he held her hand, or wrapped his arm round her, or kissed her goodnight, she'd wanted him a little more. And, if she was honest with herself, it was why she'd agreed to go back to his flat for a nightcap. She hadn't wanted a drink. She'd wanted *him*.

Common sense nudged its way in. Just. 'I don't have any condoms,' she said.

'I do.' There was a slight flush of colour along his cheekbones. 'Not because I'm taking you for granted, and not because I sleep around, because I don't actually sleep with that many women—but I'm a midwife. I know it's sensible to be prepared for every situation.'

This first time was going to be messy and hopeless; they'd have no idea what each other liked, or where each other liked being touched or kissed or stroked. Part of her really didn't want to disappoint him. But the greater part of her couldn't resist him. 'OK. But I'm rusty,' she warned.

'That doesn't matter.' He held her gaze. 'Are you sure about this?'

'I'm sure.'

'Then,' he said, 'let me show you the rest of the flat.'

She let him lead her through to his bedroom, where the curtains were already drawn.

The room was small but impeccably neat. A double bed with a black wrought-iron headboard took up most of the space, and the duvet cover was in masculine shades of blue and grey.

He cupped her face in his hands and kissed her. 'Is there a clever fastening?' he asked, looking at her little black dress.

'There's a zip at the back,' she said, turning round.

He undid the zip, drawing it down slowly, his fingers brushing against her skin as he revealed it. Then he kissed the nape of her neck, his mouth moving slowly down her spine, and she gasped. 'That feels amazing.'

He turned her round to face him again; she slipped the dress off and folded it neatly before placing it on the floor.

He sucked in a breath. 'You're gorgeous. Stunning.'

'Thank you.' She felt the colour pool in her face. 'I feel ridiculously shy. I think it's because you're wearing too much.'

'Do something about it, then,' he invited.

She undid the buttons of his shirt; the cotton was soft but his skin was even softer. Her fingers shook slightly as she undid the buttons, and she fumbled a couple of them.

He stole a kiss. 'OK?' His eyes were full of concern.

She nodded. 'Just...it's been a while.'

'That's fine,' he said, brushing the pad of his thumb over her lower lip, and her mouth tingled with anticipation. 'I'm going to enjoy you exploring me.'

'I'm going to enjoy you exploring me, too,' she whispered, and pushed the soft material of his shirt over his shoulders. She liked the definition of the muscles on his arms and his pecs. 'Do a twirl for me?'

'A twirl?' He looked surprised.

'So I can admire your muscles.'

A corner of his mouth quirked. 'I'm not exactly the sort who spends hours pumping iron.' But he turned in a circle anyway, letting her look at him.

He really was beautiful. If she'd been artistic, she would've wanted to sculpt him.

'Your shoulders are beautiful,' she said.

'Thank you.' He kissed her lightly. 'Your turn for the twirl.'

'Me? But…'

'You made me do it,' he reminded her, 'so it's only fair.'

Feeling a bit gauche, shy and awkward, she turned in a circle.

'You have beautiful curves,' he said. 'Take your hair down for me?' He gave her a rueful smile. 'Horribly cheesy, but I'd love to see your hair loose.'

And that admission was so sweet and charming. She liked the fact that he could laugh at himself. Once she'd loosened her hair and put the pins on his dressing table, he said, 'And another twirl?'

'You first,' she said.

It was silly and teenagery and…*fun*. She couldn't remember the last time she'd done anything like this. And she was still laughing when he drew her back into his arms and kissed her.

She wasn't sure which of them removed which item of clothing after that, but the next thing she knew he'd pushed his duvet aside, picked her up and laid her down on the bed. The mattress was comfortable and the fat pillows were even more comfortable, and she luxuriated against them.

He caught a breath. 'Do you have any idea how gorgeous you look like that?'

The compliment felt genuine and it boosted her confidence to the point where she could smile at him. 'Thank you.'

She felt the mattress dip as he joined her, and turned to face him; she kissed him and stroked his hair back off his forehead.

He deepened the kiss, then shifted so he could dip his head and nuzzle the hollows of her collarbones.

She'd almost forgotten what it felt like to make love; part of her was nervous, but she remembered what he said about not overthinking it and pushed the thoughts away. Instead, she concentrated on the way he made her feel, the way his mouth and his hands were skimming across her skin and coaxing a response from her.

She tipped her head back against the pillows as he shifted back down the bed, kissing the hollow beneath her ankle bone and then stroking, kissing, teasing his way upwards; she dragged in a breath as he kissed his way along her inner thigh, and she couldn't help herself sliding her hands into his hair as his tongue stroked along her sex.

Need and desire spiralled within her.

'Now,' she whispered.

He reached across to the beside cabinet, took a foil packet from a drawer and ripped it open, then slid on the condom and pushed into her.

And then he stopped. 'OK?' he asked.

She appreciated the way he was holding himself back and thinking of her needs first, knowing it was a long while since she'd had sex and realising that it might feel strange.

'Very OK,' she said, and reached up to kiss him.

Then he began to move.

Rebecca had forgotten that it could feel like this. She couldn't think of anything now except the way he made her feel, the pleasure coiling tighter and tighter within her, and then that blissful moment of release flooding through her. She felt his body surge against hers and knew he'd reached his own release.

He withdrew. 'I'm going to deal with the condom, but please don't go anywhere,' he said, 'because I really want a cuddle.'

It was unexpectedly sweet and made her like him even more.

She snuggled back under the covers and waited for him. He returned with a towel wrapped round his waist, and she grinned. 'How can you be shy after what we just did?'

He grinned back. 'I'm not shy, but I was thinking about my manners. I didn't want to come back in and wave my bits around at you like a caveman.'

'How do you know cavemen waved their bits around?'

'A wild guess,' he said; then he dropped the towel and climbed back into bed with her.

It was nice just to lie there with her head pillowed on his shoulder and his arm holding her close, her own arm wrapped round his waist.

It felt warm and sweet, having Rebecca cuddled into him. There was no need to talk, and the silence between them was restful rather than awkward. If he was honest with himself, Nathaniel didn't want her to go, but he knew she couldn't stay the night.

As if she was reading his mind, she twisted her face round to drop a kiss on his shoulder. 'I really need to be getting back. Sas is babysitting and Jasmine's got her swimming lesson tomorrow.'

'I've had three cocktails tonight so I can't drive you home myself—but I know a reliable taxi firm,' he said. 'I'll call them for you. If you want a shower first, you're welcome to use anything in the bathroom and I'll grab you a fresh towel.'

'Thanks. That would be good.'

He called the taxi and got dressed while she

was in the bathroom, and made a fuss of the cat while he waited for her to finish getting ready. When she joined him in his living room, she was fully dressed.

'The taxi will be here in five minutes,' he said. 'They just texted me.' He paused. 'I'll see you home.'

'You don't have to do that.' She shook her head. 'You said yourself they were reliable.'

'Yeah, but I want to snatch a few more minutes with you.' He was aware of how needy that made him sound, and groaned. 'That's pathetic. Anyone would think I was twelve, not thirty-four.'

'Actually, it's really cute.' She stole a kiss. 'And I kind of like the idea of you holding my hand in the back seat of a car, all the way home.'

The reality was even better. They didn't need to talk; they just sat with his arm round her, her head on his shoulder, and their hands linked on their laps.

Finally, the taxi pulled up outside her house.

'Thank you for an amazing evening,' she said softly.

'Thank *you*.' He kissed her lightly. 'I guess I'll see you at work. But maybe we can steal some time together next week.'

'I'm on an early on Wednesday,' she said.

'Me, too. If you can get a babysitter, we'll work out where we can go between now and then.'

'I'd like that.' She kissed him. 'Sweet dreams.'

He knew they would be. Because they'd be of her.

He asked the taxi driver to wait until she was inside before driving him back to his flat.

When he walked through the door, Leo greeted him with a quizzical purr.

'Yes, Leo, I had a lovely night,' Nathaniel told the cat. 'I like her. I *really* like her. She's special.'

And he just hoped she was starting to feel the same way about him.

CHAPTER TEN

IN THE MIDDLE of Wednesday afternoon, Rebecca was called down to the Emergency Department. 'Molly Davidson's waiting in the cubicle,' Ellie, the charge nurse, said. 'We've done urine and blood tests, and we've stabilised her with oxygen and fluids and given her some pain relief. She's thirty-four, and she's had single-sided abdominal pain for a couple of days now but assumed she was just having a worse than usual attack of endometriosis.'

Oh, no. This sounded familiar.

Rebecca damped down the memories. Not now. 'Did you do a pregnancy test?' she asked.

'Yes, and it's positive,' Ellie said. 'The baby wasn't planned and her periods aren't that regular, but we've worked out she's probably about seven weeks. She hasn't had any bleeding, but she felt a bit faint this morning, she's had shoulder-tip pain and she collapsed at work an hour ago. One of her colleagues called an ambulance, and I asked you to come down because I think we're looking at an ectopic pregnancy and a ruptured tube.'

'Sadly, it sounds as if you're spot on,' Rebecca said. And she knew exactly what that felt like.

'I've got the portable scanner on its way,' Ellie said. 'And we've called her partner. He's coming in now.'

'Perfect. Thank you,' Rebecca said.

'Let me introduce you,' Ellie said, and led Rebecca over to the cubicle. 'Miss Davidson, this is Dr Hart. I'm going to leave her to have a chat with you. Is that OK?'

At Molly's nod, Rebecca thanked Ellie as she left the cubicle. 'Ellie's filled me in on how you're feeling right now. I need to do a scan to confirm it, but it sounds to me as if you have an ectopic pregnancy. That means the embryo got stuck in your fallopian tube instead of travelling all the way down to your womb, so the egg's growing in the wrong place.'

It was so easy to say. All neat and tidy and fixable. But Rebecca also knew how it felt: a pain sharper than labour, and then the grief afterwards for a baby that didn't have a chance. The fear that things might never be OK again.

In her case, it was the baby she and Lucas

hadn't known about. An unexpected last gift she hadn't been able to keep.

'I'm going to give you a scan but, because you're in such pain, I'm pretty sure your fallopian tube has ruptured and you're going to need an operation for me to repair it,' she said.

Molly's face was white. 'An operation.'

'I'll do it under general anaesthetic,' Rebecca explained, 'so you'll be asleep when it's carried out. I'll do my best to repair the tube, but if I can't then I'll need to remove it to stop the bleeding and to keep you safe.' Which was exactly what had happened to her.

'I had no idea I was pregnant. We tried for a couple of years and it never happened, because of my endometriosis, and we're on the waiting list for IVF.' Molly looked distraught. 'Isn't there anything you can do to save the baby?'

Rebecca took her hand. 'I'm so sorry. The only place an embryo can grow and get the nutrients it needs to survive is in your womb. Your health is uppermost for us now, so surgery is the only option. But the good news is I can do it by keyhole surgery, so you'll be able to go home in a day or so.'

Just then, Ellie came back into the cubicle. 'Molly, your partner's here.'

'Dan!' Molly collapsed into tears again while her partner hugged her.

Rebecca slipped out to grab tissues and a cup of water for her patient.

'Here. These might help,' she said gently.

'Dr Hart was saying that I need keyhole surgery,' Molly said.

'What does that mean?' Dan asked.

'It's still done under a general anaesthetic, but the incisions are much smaller so Molly will recover from the operation quicker,' Rebecca explained. 'Once you're under, Molly, I'll make some small incisions in your stomach and put a small flexible tube inside you which has fibre optic lights and a camera on the end. It sends me images of your abdomen so I can operate. Hopefully I'll be able to repair your fallopian tube, but as I said if I can't repair it, I'll have to remove it. Then I'll minimise any bleeding and stitch you up. It'll take between thirty minutes and an hour.'

'But if you have to remove the tube completely, does that mean I won't ever be able to have a baby?' Molly asked.

'Even with one tube, you'll still have a good chance of conceiving naturally—roughly six in ten—though it's more likely that you might have an ectopic pregnancy in future,' Rebecca said. Stats she'd dully listened to her own surgeon telling her, too; it had felt as if she were hearing it all underwater, at slow speed, the words not going in.

Jasmine dearly wanted a little sister, she knew. But even if this thing with Nathaniel worked out, that ectopic pregnancy would come back to haunt her. She might not be able to give Nathaniel a child and Jasmine a sibling. And what then?

'I know you said you were on the waiting list for IVF, but I'd suggest giving yourself three months to recover before you start trying for a baby again. If it happens before you have the IVF treatment, I'd advise you to come and see us pretty much as soon as you know you're pregnant, so we can monitor you and keep a close eye on you.'

Molly bit her lip. 'Is it likely it'd be ectopic again, if I fell pregnant?'

'An ectopic pregnancy is more common if you've had one already,' Rebecca said, trying to damp down her memories again—her patient needed reassurance, not a meltdown. 'But I want you to know that there's still a good chance that it would be a normal pregnancy, next time.'

'If it was another ectopic pregnancy, would I lose my other tube?'

'Not necessarily,' Rebecca said. 'It depends what sort of symptoms you're having. Sometimes we just wait and see, and the pregnancy ends itself naturally. Sometimes we can give you medication to stop the pregnancy growing and avoid surgery.'

'Can't you give her medication instead of doing surgery today?' Dan asked.

'No. I'm afraid that only works if a woman has only mild symptoms, and I'm pretty sure there's a rupture—I'll know more when I've done the scan.'

Just as she said it, the portable scanner arrived.

And the scan itself confirmed everything that Rebecca and Ellie had suspected. 'I'm sorry,' Rebecca said. 'You've got internal bleeding, Molly, so I'm going to need to take you to Theatre.'

'Why did it happen?' Dan asked.

'We don't necessarily know why,' Rebecca told him. 'If you've had previous surgery on your fallopian tubes or a previous ectopic pregnancy, it increases the risk—but, in more than half the cases, there's no reason. Sometimes it's caused by pelvic inflammatory disease, sometimes there's a hormonal imbalance, or sometimes it's the way the egg develops.' She squeezed Molly's hand. 'It's not something you could've prevented, so don't blame yourself.' Though she knew what that devastation felt like. Even though her doctor's training told her otherwise, she'd had a moment when she'd wondered if she'd done something wrong or all the stress of losing Lucas had caused it. She knew it wasn't true, but it hadn't done much to ease the misery. 'It's absolutely *not* your fault. I'm going to introduce you to the anaesthetist, and then I'll scrub up and we'll get you into Theatre. Dan, I'm afraid you can't go in to Theatre with Molly, but you can be with her until she leaves, and wait in the waiting room.'

The operation was a success; once Molly was round from the anaesthetic, Rebecca scrubbed out and took Dan to see her in the recovery room.

'Did you manage to save the tube?' was Molly's first question.

'I'm sorry, I'm afraid I couldn't,' Rebecca said. 'But the good news is your other tube looked healthy.'

A tear dripped down Molly's cheek. 'We're on the waiting list for IVF. We didn't think I could get pregnant naturally. And...' She choked. 'I can't believe I actually got pregnant and then this happened.'

'I'm so sorry,' Rebecca said. 'But you do still have a good chance of having a baby in the future.' The words echoed hollowly in her head. It was one of the things she worried about with

Nathaniel. What if he wanted children and she couldn't have them?

'What happens now?' Dan asked.

'When the anaesthetist is happy, we'll take Molly up to the ward—the gynae ward, not the maternity ward,' Rebecca added swiftly. 'You might be in a bit of discomfort later, Molly, either in your shoulder tip or your abdomen, but we can give you pain relief for that, and the nurses will be there to help you.'

'I lost the baby,' Molly whispered. 'And I wanted a baby so much.'

'I know. We both did. But it'll be better next time,' Dan said, holding her tightly. 'It's going to be fine.'

Rebecca felt completely helpless. Their dreams had been smashed, and there was nothing she could do to fix it. All she could do now was to focus on the practical stuff. It was what she'd ended up doing herself—focusing on the practical stuff. Organising a funeral. Looking after her toddler. Putting one foot in front of the other and keeping going.

'The stitches should dissolve within a couple of weeks, but don't put any talc or moisturiser on the wound. If you spot any redness or swelling once you go home, go to see your GP,' she said. 'The scars will hardly be visible in a couple of months.'

'When can I go home?' Molly asked.

'Tomorrow, if you feel up to it. Make sure you rest for at least the next couple of weeks, take some gentle exercise and avoid heavy lifting, and if you feel up to it you'll be able to go back to work in two to four weeks. Come back and see me for a check-up in six weeks, and if you're worried about anything I'm here.' She took a deep breath. 'I know this is horrible for both of you. I can organise some counselling, and I'd recommend getting in touch with a support group. It helps to talk to people who've been through it, too—people who've come out the other side and will have some practical ideas to help both of you through the heartache.' She almost—*almost*—told them she'd been through it herself and she was talking from experience, but right at that moment she needed to calm her emotions down again.

'Thank you,' they said, but she could see the devastation in their faces and it made her feel horrible. Just as bad as she'd felt when she'd lost the baby. And the guilt she'd felt later at thinking that maybe it had been for the best—how, as a young widow, could she have coped with a toddler and a newborn? And, if Lucas had survived the crash, their marriage definitely wouldn't have survived all the changes and compromises that a second child would have brought.

By the time Rebecca went back up to her office, she was drained. All she wanted to do was go home and hug her little girl tightly. She was so, so lucky to have Jasmine.

And she really couldn't face her night out with Nathaniel tonight. She needed to rebalance her equilibrium. Going out felt so trivial, so pointless, when such serious things were going on in other people's lives.

Nathaniel had already finished his shift and gone home, so she texted him.

Sorry. Need to call off tonight. Had a rough shift. It's me, not you.

That sounded as if she was dumping him, and she didn't want to give him that impression. Though she didn't want to explain either.

She added,

Maybe we can go out some other time. Just not tonight. R x

Nathaniel looked at the text on his phone. He wasn't aware of any difficult cases on the ward today, but maybe someone from the Emergency Department had asked Rebecca to treat a patient. He knew she'd been in Theatre when he'd left.

Theatre, and a rough shift. It sounded as if the baby hadn't made it—the kind of case they all found hard to deal with. He hated to think she was so upset about work but would have to go home and pretend that everything was completely fine, for Jasmine's sake.

Maybe there was something he could do to help.

The florists were all closed by now, but the big supermarket round the corner from him had a decent range of flowers. He chose a large bunch of bright sunflowers, waited until he was pretty sure Jasmine would be asleep, and drove round to Rebecca's house.

Ringing the doorbell might wake the little girl, so he texted her.

Got a moment? On your front doorstep.

Two minutes later, the front door opened.

'Nathaniel, I—' she began.

'I'm not staying,' he cut in. 'I know you've had a tough day. So I just wanted to give you a hug and bring you these, because I wanted to make your day a little bit better.' He handed her the sunflowers.

She looked at them, then him, and tears spilled over her lashes.

He couldn't leave her like this. Gently, he put his arms around her and ushered her back into the house. He closed the front door behind them and held her tightly, cradling her head on his shoulder and letting her cry.

Eventually, she lifted her head. 'I'm sorry for sobbing all over you. I hate these kind of days,' she whispered. 'The sort of days where I can't make a difference.'

'What happened?'

'The Emergency Department called me down to a patient who'd collapsed and they thought it might be an ectopic pregnancy. She had a ruptured tube. The baby wasn't planned, but she really wanted it—she thought she might have to have IVF treatment before she could have a child.' She shook her head. 'I couldn't save the baby or the tube. The poor woman and her partner were both devastated.'

He winced. 'That's hard. But you did make a difference, Rebecca. You operated and you saved her life. And you know as well as I do that you can't save an ectopic pregnancy.'

'Intellectually, I know that. But emotionally…' She dragged in a breath. 'I had an ectopic pregnancy. After Lucas died. I didn't even know I was pregnant. I'd only just started organising the funeral, and suddenly I had this terrible pain and collapsed. So I know exactly what that poor woman went through today.'

He held her closer. 'Is this the first ectopic you've had to deal with since?'

She shook her head. 'But it got to me today. Jasmine was telling me this morning over breakfast that her best friend at nursery is having a little sister. And then she asked me if she could have a little sister, too.' Rebecca swallowed hard. 'I managed to distract her, but it made me think. There's no guarantee I could have another child. The tube was ruptured, so I lost it. There I was this afternoon, telling Molly Davidson that she still had a good chance of having another baby, but...'

He knew what she was trying to tell him. That she came with complications. That, even if their relationship worked out, she might not be able to give him a child. And he'd told her he wanted a family.

He stroked her hair. 'None of us knows what the future holds. And if you want another child and your fallopian tube is a problem, you can always consider fostering or adoption.'

She looked at him, and he could see the question in her eyes. What did *he* want?

He'd always planned to have kids with Angie. After she'd dumped him, he'd vowed to be happy being godfather to his best friend's daughter and uncle to Charlotte's children.

But at that point he'd told himself he wouldn't have another serious relationship. Now... Everything was different. Rebecca might just be the one worth taking the risk with. Yet now she was telling him that having more children might not be a possibility for her.

He needed some time to process this. So he held her close again. 'You've had a horrible day, but your patient is still alive, thanks to you. If you hadn't operated, with a ruptured fallopian tube she could've bled out and died,' he said. 'Focus on the good stuff.'

'I'm sorry I called off our date at the last minute.'

'Nobody would want to go out, in your shoes. I'm not taking it personally,' he reassured her. Was that the way Lucas would have reacted?

He stroked her hair. 'I just wanted to make you feel a bit better, that's all. So I brought you some sunshine in flower form, and the plan was for me to give you a hug and go.'

'Thank you.' She pulled back slightly so she could look him in the eye. 'A bit of me wants to tell you to stay.'

'But Jasmine's asleep, you have work tomorrow—and we have all the time in the world,' he said. He couldn't resist stealing a kiss, brushing his mouth lightly over hers. 'It can wait. So can our date. And it'll be all the sweeter when it happens.'

There was a glimmer of a smile through her tears. 'Yeah.'

'You're a good woman, Rebecca Hart, and you're an amazing doctor. Don't you forget it.' He kissed her again. 'I'll see you tomorrow. Sleep tight. And if you're awake in the middle of the night, feeling miserable, call me.'

'I can't do that. You'll be asleep.'

He smiled. 'And you're one of the people I won't mind waking me. If you need me, I'm there.'

'That's...' She shook her head, as if lost for words, and stroked his face. 'You're the nicest man I know, Nathaniel Jones.'

'You're not so shabby yourself.' One last kiss, and he dragged himself away before he begged her to let him stay.

Because Rebecca Hart was worth the wait.

CHAPTER ELEVEN

On Thursday morning, Nathaniel thought about calling Rebecca before his shift; but he knew she'd be busy with the morning routine of getting Jasmine ready. It would be better to text her, so she could pick it up at a time that suited her.

How are you? Xx

The reply came quicker than he'd expected.

Better. And thank you for yesterday. xx

My pleasure.

He paused.

What shift are you on tomorrow? Xx

Late. xx

Perfect.

If you're not busy, I could do with some female advice. Involves shopping. xx

Shopping? Xx

Something to cheer up a grumpy, very pregnant and overdue sister. xx

You're on. Meet you at the Tube station after the nursery run? Nine fifteen OK? Xx

Nine fifteen it is. xx

Nathaniel's path didn't cross Rebecca's at work that day—he was in clinic and she was in Theatre—but he met her at the Tube station as planned on Friday morning.

'Hey.' To his relief, she hadn't gone shy on him as she greeted him with a hug.

'So what do you have in mind to cheer your sister up?' she asked.

'Starting with flowers; something girly—which is where you come in; and I thought I'd take her freshly squeezed orange juice and a bit of organic carrot cake and spend some time with her,' he said. 'There's no obligation for you to do any more than the shopping—and I'm very grateful for that—but if you'd like to come and visit her with me, you'd be very welcome.'

'I'd like that,' she said.

Funny, he'd always loathed shopping with Angela, dragging around the shops while she dithered and looked at everything six times before going back to the first shop again. But with Rebecca it was easy. She steered him into a shop which specialised in freshly made toiletries with hypoallergenic, natural ingredients. 'When I was pregnant, the thing I hated was getting puffy feet. So I think a foot-soak and foot cream would be the perfect treat,' she said.

The assistant wrapped the toiletries in a pretty fabric wrapper for him. Once they'd picked up flowers, cake and juice, they were at Charlotte's house by half-past ten.

'For you,' Nathaniel said, and gave his sister a hug. 'You look as if you had a rough night,'

'I couldn't settle.' She wrinkled her nose. 'I must've eaten something that disagreed with me yesterday and gave me indigestion. I've been getting twinges all morning.'

Nathaniel and Rebecca exchanged a glance.

'Charlotte, your due date was last week. Are you sure you're not having contractions?' Nathaniel asked.

'Of course I'm sure.' She rolled her eyes. 'I had Braxton-Hicks last week, and they felt a lot stronger than this. I just ate something that gave me a bit of indigestion, that's all.'

'Have you taken anything for it?' Rebecca asked.

Charlotte nodded. 'That horribly chalky stuff the pharmacist said is safe for pregnant women to take for heartburn.'

'And it hasn't helped?' Nathaniel asked.

'What is this, twenty questions?' Charlotte asked irritably.

'He's just being a concerned big brother,' Rebecca said, clearly trying to pour oil on troubled waters. 'I'd ask the same, if you were my sister. And I'd also ask if you had any back pain.'

'A little bit,' Charlotte admitted, 'but probably because I couldn't get comfortable last night so I must've lain awkwardly. I walked it off round the kitchen.'

Nathaniel exchanged another glance with Rebecca. The more his sister was saying, the more it sounded as if she was in labour. And she wasn't usually the irritable sort.

'Let me put your flowers in water for you,' Rebecca offered. 'Tell me where you keep your vases.'

'Kitchen cupboard. Come through,' Charlotte said.

Then she stopped in the doorway. 'Oh!'

'OK, sis?' Nathaniel asked.

'Stupid pelvic floor.' She grimaced. 'Even though I did all the exercises, it feels as if I've wet myself. I *hate* this. Look, I'm just going to the bathroom to clean myself up.'

'Charlotte, please don't think I'm interfering,' Rebecca said, 'but have you thought that might've been your waters breaking rather than a leak from your bladder?'

'They'd better not. Robyn isn't—ow!' Charlotte grabbed the doorway.

'With my professional hat on, I'd say your indigestion was the first stage of labour,' Rebecca said, 'and your waters have broken. Would you let me examine you, or would you rather we called Robyn and an ambulance now?'

'You can examine me if you really want to, but I'm not in la—' Charlotte doubled over.

'I'm calling Robyn,' Nathaniel said, and speed-dialled his sister-in-law while Rebecca helped Charlotte over to the kitchen table and spread clean tea towels over it before helping Charlotte up to examine her. 'Robyn? I'm at your place with Rebecca. We think Charlotte's in labour.'

'Oh, my God. I'm coming now. Are you taking her to hospital?'

'Are we taking her to hospital?' He looked at Rebecca, who shook her head. 'No. We're calling an ambulance. I'll keep you posted on what's happening.'

'I'm leaving now. I'm getting a taxi. Tell Charlotte I love her.'

'I will,' he promised, then called the ambulance while he grabbed a pile of clean towels from the airing cupboard.

'Why have you got towels?' Charlotte wanted to know.

'Just call it a midwife's instinct,' he said.

'You think I'm having the baby *now*? No way. They said in antenatal classes that a first labour takes an average of twelve hours, and those were the first contractions I felt,' Charlotte protested.

They might've been the first ones his sister had felt, but he was pretty sure they weren't her first actual contractions. And he wasn't sure how to break it to her that some babies took an awful lot less time than twelve hours to arrive.

'When did the ambulance say they'd be here?' Rebecca asked.

'Twenty minutes,' he told her. 'Robyn says she loves you.'

'I hate to tell you this, Charlotte,' Rebecca said gently, 'but I've been timing your contractions. I agree with Nathaniel. I don't think you'll make it to hospital.'

'But I'm not in labour,' Charlotte protested, shaking her head. 'Ow!'

'Your baby has other ideas. I reckon my niece is planning on a fast labour and a home birth,' Nathaniel said. 'So having an obstetrician and a midwife with you might be useful.'

'A home birth? What, right now?' Charlotte went white. 'But—I can't. Not without Robyn here.'

'Robyn's on her way and I'm keeping her posted,' Nathaniel said. 'In the meantime, did you hire that TENS machine and is it in your labour bag?'

'No. You made me pack that bag weeks ago,' she grumbled. 'I was going to pick up the machine tomorrow.'

No pain relief, then. But there was an ambulance on the way and an obstetrician right beside him. They could do this.

'Let me examine you again,' Rebecca said.

Nathaniel held his sister's hand while Rebecca examined her.

'Eight centimetres dilated,' she said. 'This baby definitely wants to make her arrival soon.'

'But I can't be,' Charlotte said.

'You've probably been in labour all night,' Rebecca said gently. 'That indigestion and backache were contractions. You just didn't feel them the way you expected to.'

'Oh, my God.' Charlotte looked shocked. 'Robyn didn't want to leave me to go to work this morning, but I chugged some of the chalky stuff and told her I'd be fine, it was just indigestion.' Her eyes filled with tears. 'I'll never forgive myself if she misses our baby being born.'

'Relax,' Nathaniel said. 'It's all going to be fine. She's on the way right now. She'll be here before the little one arrives.'

'And we'll be here to support you and help you breathe until she gets here,' Rebecca said, exchanging a glance with Nathaniel.

Between them, they encouraged Charlotte to breathe and to walk around the kitchen.

'I'm going to put the heating on and close the doors and windows, so it's nice and warm in here for the baby,' Nathaniel said. 'Which room do you want to give birth in?'

'I'm going to make a right mess of the carpet,' Charlotte said.

Nathaniel smiled. 'No, you won't. If you want to go into the living room, I'll put some bin liners down to protect the carpet, a sheet over that, and some towels so it's comfy for you. Give me a few minutes, and we'll sort it.'

'Light a candle so you've got nice scent in the air, and put some music on—you don't have to throw your entire birth plan out of the window,' Rebecca added.

He busied himself making the living room comfortable for his sister, then came back in to help Rebecca support her through to the living room.

'Squeeze my hand whenever you need to,' he directed. 'Whatever makes you comfortable. You've got this. Just a few more minutes until Robyn's here. You can hold on. You can do *anything* for just five minutes.'

It reminded Rebecca of the way he'd talked her through the abseil. She'd thought then how good he'd be with mums going through an uncomplicated labour, and this proved her point.

She was timing the contractions, which were getting closer together.

'How far apart?' Nathaniel mouthed.

'Two minutes,' she mouthed back.

Charlotte puffed. 'I can't…'

'It's fine, sweetheart. Tell me what you need,' Rebecca encouraged gently.

Charlotte's face reddened. 'If I do a poo in front of my little brother…'

'It won't matter in the slightest. Forget the fact he's your little brother. He's a qualified midwife and he's really good at what he does. He's seen it all before and so have I,' Rebecca reassured her. 'We don't care about any of that. We just want you to be comfortable and relaxed.'

'Breathe for me,' Nathaniel said. 'Then start to bear down when you need to push.'

'OK.' Charlotte was close to tears.

Just then, there was a rattle at the door and Robyn rushed in. 'Charlotte!'

'I didn't think you'd make it.' A fat tear rolled down Charlotte's cheek.

'She's here now, so let Nathaniel and me examine you,' Rebecca said. 'Robyn's taking over hand-holding duties.'

She quickly examined Charlotte. 'Ten centimetres,' she said in a low voice.

'Remember your class about birth positions?' Nathaniel asked.

Charlotte nodded. 'I was going to kneel.'

'That's fine. I'll get you a chair,' Nathaniel said.

Once he'd brought in the chair, he and Robyn supported Charlotte so she was kneeling and holding on to the chair.

'I need to push,' Charlotte said.

'Breathe, and we'll be here to guide the baby,' Rebecca said. She and Nathaniel knelt behind Charlotte, and she examined Charlotte. 'Crowning,' she mouthed to Nathaniel. 'Charlotte, I want you to stop pushing. I need you to blow little short breaths out of your mouth.'

'Just like we practised,' Robyn said, and demonstrated.

The head was born slowly and gently.

'Another push with that next contraction,' Nathaniel said. 'You've got this, Charlotte. Nearly there.'

Another push, and the baby's head turned to the side.

'Now do some more of those short breaths,' Rebecca directed, while Nathaniel supported the baby's head and checked that the cord wasn't wrapped round her neck. 'That's brilliant. Keep going.'

'Another push,' Nathaniel said, and the baby's first shoulder slipped out. A second, and the other shoulder came out and the baby slithered into Nathaniel's hands.

'She's here!' Nathaniel said. 'And she's perfect.'

The baby cried, to Rebecca's relief, then started to pink up nicely. 'Let me wipe her face,' she said.

Robyn handed her a clean cloth, and Rebecca wiped the baby's face and wrapped her in a clean sheet.

'We want to keep the baby warm, so we're going to help you shift round, Charlotte. Then I'm going to put the baby on your chest and wrap a towel over both of you,' Rebecca said.

'What about the cord?' Robyn asked, looking anxious.

'It's long enough to let the baby be on Charlotte's chest, and hopefully the ambulance crew will be here with clamps and sterile scissors very shortly,' Nathaniel said. 'Though we might have to improvise.'

'If you can put a hat on the baby, Robyn, that'd be great,' Rebecca said. 'Charlotte, let the baby nuzzle your breast—it'll help your body produce the hormones so you can deliver the placenta more easily.'

Just as soon as Charlotte was settled with the baby, the doorbell went.

Rebecca went to answer it and led the ambulance crew into the living room. 'I'm afraid the baby had other plans, so you've missed the exciting bit,' she said with a smile, 'but we could do with some sterile clamps and scissors.'

Robyn cut the cord, and Nathaniel helped Charlotte to deliver the placenta.

'Congratulations, both of you,' Rebecca said, smiling as Charlotte and Robyn cuddled their baby.

Delivering babies was one thing; delivering his niece was beyond anything he'd ever experienced, and Nathaniel was moved to tears.

'Hey, Uncle Nathaniel. I'd better get to work. I'll call the boss on the way and get some cover for you,' Rebecca whispered, and gave him a hug.

'Cover?' He looked at her, too dazed to take in what she was saying.

'You just delivered your sister's baby.'

'*We* delivered her,' Nathaniel corrected.

'In your shoes, I'd want to stay here with my family for a bit.'

'I do,' he admitted.

'Leave it to me and I'll sort it out.' She smiled at him. 'I'd better be off. See you later.'

'Thank you for everything you did. You were amazing.'

'*Charlotte* was amazing,' she said. 'Go be with your family. They'll need you to take them in to be checked over properly.' She hugged Robyn and Charlotte. 'Congratulations. Your daughter's beautiful.'

'Delilah,' Robyn said.

'Great name.'

After Rebecca had gone, Nathaniel took Charlotte, Robyn and Delilah in to their local hospital for a check-up with their own midwifery team.

It was while he was in the waiting area that it hit him. Everyone around him was part of a family. There were couples on their own, glowing with the thrill of their first child. Couples with smaller children, clearly wanting their older child to be there for the scan. Single mums with a sister or a mum or a friend supporting them.

In his own department, he saw families of all shapes and sizes every day. He'd thought by now that he would have children of his own. If it hadn't been for falling off that roof, he would've been married to Angela, and with luck they would've had babies.

But all the dreams had shattered into smaller pieces than his bones, after his fall. It had taken only days for Angela to decide he wasn't enough for her. So what made him think he'd be enough for Rebecca?

Yes, they'd been getting on well, and he was starting to fall in love with the serious obstetrician who had a sweet, playful side she kept hidden. And yes, he could imagine making a family with her and Jasmine. They could be a unit, just like his sister with Robyn and Delilah.

That was what he wanted. A family. Himself, Rebecca, Jasmine and maybe a little brother or sister.

But what if it wasn't what *she* wanted?

The voice in the back of his head—the one he tried so hard to silence—wouldn't shut up. It kept telling him he was a fraud. He hadn't been enough for Angie, and he hadn't made any of his subsequent relationships work—because he hadn't wanted to commit his heart, only to have it broken again. What if he wasn't good enough for Rebecca, either?

She'd already been in one relationship where she hadn't been happy. She'd had the courage to plan to leave Lucas; maybe in a few months, when she realised Nathaniel wasn't enough for her, she'd leave him, too.

And that, he realised, would shatter his heart even more than Angie had.

So maybe he should stop now. Save himself the heartbreak.

It took him ages to find the right words.

Thank you for what you did today. I've been thinking—I think it's better that you and I are just good friends. Sorry to let you down. N x

He stared at the message for a while, and finally hit 'send'.

If only things could've been different.

But they weren't. He would never be enough for her.

Rebecca stared at the words on her phone screen.

Thank you for what you did today. I've been thinking—I think it's better that you and I are just good friends. Sorry to let you down. N x

What?

He was ending it?

But...they'd delivered his sister's baby together. She'd met his family and got on well with them. He'd met Jasmine and she'd adored him. They'd been planning for him to meet her mum and dad and Saskia.

Why would he end it?

She didn't understand. Everything had been going fine.

Or maybe she'd been fooling herself all along. Maybe she'd made exactly the same mistake that she'd made with Lucas, and she'd fallen for someone who didn't want commitment.

Given that Nathaniel could end this so casually, by text rather than bothering to tell her to her face, he clearly thought she and Jasmine were easily dispensable.

And it hurt. It hurt so much.

It made her ribs feel as if they'd just cracked, because her heart had swollen in misery, and her skin felt tight and prickly. She'd been close to declaring her feelings, and she'd actually let him into Jasmine's life as well as her own: and this was how he'd treated her. As if she was worthless.

Just like Lucas had made her feel.

Well, she wasn't going to beg someone to

love her when he clearly didn't. She'd been there, done that—and it seemed that she'd been stupid enough to do it all over again.

This was the last time she'd make that particular mistake.

And she'd have a quiet word with the head of department to see if she could change her shifts, so her path wouldn't cross that much with Nathaniel's in the future.

He'd made it clear that he didn't want to discuss it, and in any case she didn't know what to say. All she could do was send back a message.

OK.

And that was it.
Over.

CHAPTER TWELVE

THANKFULLY NATHANIEL WAS on duty over the weekend and Rebecca wasn't, so she didn't have to face him. She managed to avoid him on the ward at the beginning of the week, but on Wednesday, she was in clinic when Amara knocked on the door. 'Dr Hart, I'm sorry to interrupt, but it's urgent.'

The midwife looked worried, and Rebecca's breath caught. What was wrong? Had something happened to Jasmine? To her parents? To her sister? 'Excuse me, please,' she said to her mum-to-be. 'I'll be back in a moment.'

She stepped outside the room. 'What's happened?' she asked.

'Jasmine's nursery rang. There's been an accident.'

Rebecca went cold all over. 'What sort of accident?'

'She fell off a climbing frame. She's been sick and she's got a headache. The ambulance is bringing her in to the Emergency Department now.'

Rebecca wrapped one arm round herself, shivering. A fall, and a head injury enough to cause symptoms. Fear flooded through her, worse than the moment when she'd had the call from the Emergency Department about Lucas. She'd gone to the hospital, waited while the team tried desperately to resuscitate him. Supposing this was the same?

Supposing her daughter, too, went to the Emergency Department and never came back?

'I need to go to her,' she said. She dragged in a breath. 'But my patient...'

'I'll get Tan to take over,' Amara said. 'It'll be fine. Jasmine will be fine, too.' She placed a hand on Rebecca's arm. 'You know it's standard procedure to take a little one with symptoms of concussion to be checked over.'

But what if it was more than just concussion? Rebecca knew the statistics: traumatic brain injuries were most common in children aged four and under. *Jasmine's age.*

Please, no.

She couldn't lose her daughter the way she'd lost Lucas, waiting for news in the Emergency Department.

She pulled herself together. Just. 'Thanks, Amara.' On autopilot, she went back into the consulting room. 'I'm sorry, Mrs Fraser. There's been an accident and I need to go to my little girl. One of my colleagues will be in to see you very shortly.' She forced herself to smile reassuringly, then headed for the Emergency Department at a run.

All she could think of was that when she'd kissed her little girl goodbye this morning at nursery it might have been the last time.

Please don't let it have been the last time.

Intellectually, she knew Amara was right: if a small child had a head injury, was sick and complained of a headache, then you would take that child to the Emergency Department to get checked over.

But what if it wasn't just concussion?

Supposing it wasn't the most likely thing that had happened to Jasmine, but the rare thing? They said that lightning didn't strike twice, but that wasn't true. Lucas had died of a head injury. Supposing their daughter did the same? Supposing it was a subdural haematoma?

The nearer she got to the Emergency Department, the more her fears grew, and the more she wished she'd called her parents or her sister to be with her. Most of the time, she could cope with being a single parent; but right now, in the middle of a crisis, she needed someone to lean on. She'd started to think that Nathaniel might be that someone. But then he'd backed away and she realised how wrong she'd been.

The receptionist did a double take when she saw Rebecca in the Emergency Department. 'I'm not used to seeing you this side of the department, Dr Hart. Is everything all right?'

No. It was very far from all right. She tried to stay calm. 'My daughter's on her way in with the paramedics. Jasmine Hart.'

'Hang on, I'll see what's happening.' The receptionist checked on the computer. 'It says here she's just been brought in and she's being assessed. Do you want one of us to take you through?'

Rebecca shook her head. 'Just tell me which bay and I'll find her.' Then she realised how snappy she must have sounded. 'Sorry. Thank you. Sorry, I didn't mean to be rude. My head's all over the place.'

The receptionist's face was kind. 'Don't worry, it's every mum's worst nightmare, being called to hospital for your little one. I hope everything goes OK.'

So did she. *Please, please, let Jasmine be OK.*

'Thank you,' she said.

'She's in Bay Four.' The receptionist buzzed her through, and Rebecca hurried to Bay Four. Jasmine, looking pale and still, was lying on the bed, and sitting next to her was Bethany French, Jasmine's key worker from the nursery.

'Mummy, my head hurts,' Jasmine whispered.

'I know, baby, but you're safe now,' Rebecca said, holding her hand. 'Everything's going to be fine. I'm here.'

'I'm so sorry,' Bethany said. 'One minute she was on the climbing frame, and the next she was on the floor. It happened so fast.' She bit her lip. 'She was sick, but she wasn't unconscious. We called 999 and when the ambulance came they decided to bring her in. I came with her so she'd have someone she knew with her and wouldn't be scared.'

'Thank you,' Rebecca said. Even though she was terrified, she couldn't let this poor woman think it was all her fault. 'And it wasn't your fault. I know what Jas is like with the climbing frame—she'd be on it all day if she could. It was an accident.'

'The doctor was here a minute ago,' Bethany said. 'You know—oh, she's here now.'

Rebecca glanced at the doctor walking in to the cubicle and almost sagged in relief. It was someone she knew: Hayley Price, one of the consultants, whose oldest child was the same age as Jasmine and went to the same nursery.

'Haze. Hello. Sorry. I'm all over the place.' She shook her head, trying to clear it. 'I'm…'

She'd never been the inarticulate sort, but right now she couldn't think straight. Panic and relief were clashing in her head, drowning everything else out.

'Hi, Rebecca,' Hayley said. 'Obviously you're frantic—anyone would be, in your shoes—but she's doing OK. We've checked her blood pressure, heart rate and respiration, and they're all fine. Her GCS is fifteen. She can't remember falling off the climbing frame, which as you know is pretty common after a bump to the head, but she didn't lose consciousness. She's got a bit of a bump, but otherwise she's fine. We've checked her pupils and her limb movements, and I'm happy with them, but I want to send her for a CT scan as a precaution because she was sick.'

'Uh-huh.' CT scan. The last CT scan Lucas had had… Fear gripped her again.

'I'm pretty sure it's simple concussion,' Hayley said gently. 'You know we're always cautious with little ones.'

'Thank you.' Rebecca reminded herself to breathe and not spiral back into panic mode.

'Can we call anyone for you?' Hayley asked.

'No. I'll ring my mum myself. But I'd like to be there for the scan.'

'Of course. Though obviously you'll need a lead apron.' Hayley looked at Rebecca. 'And from your own Emergency Department training you know the rules.'

That a parent could go in with their children for a CT scan, unless the mum happened to be pregnant. This was obviously Hayley's way of asking the question without breaching her privacy. 'I do, and it's fine,' Rebecca confirmed.

'Can I come, too?' Bethany asked.

'If that's OK with you, Rebecca?' Hayley asked.

'Yes.' Rebecca thought Bethany could do with some reassurance, plus it would be good to have someone waiting with her. 'I'll call my mum while you take Bethany through the consent and privacy stuff, Hayley,' she said.

She stepped into the corridor and called her mum. Caroline, as always, was unflappable. 'It's probably a precaution. I'll drive over— if she's allowed home, you'll need transport with a child seat.' And Rebecca's parents kept a spare child seat for the car at their house.

'Thanks, Mum.'

'She's going to be fine, Bec. It's not going to be like Lucas,' Caroline added softly. 'I'll be with you soon.'

The CT scan seemed to take for ever, but finally they were back in the Emergency Department, Caroline had arrived, and Rebecca was holding Jasmine's hand and reassuring her.

'Good news. It's clear,' Hayley said when she came back into their cubicle.

Clear. *Not* the subdural haematoma Rebecca had half-convinced herself it was.

Relief flooded through her so fast that, if she hadn't been sitting down, she would've fallen.

'I know you know what to look out for, but it's always different when it's one of your own,' Hayley said, 'so I'm giving you the head injuries leaflet to take home. It's an awful lot easier to look at something written down than to rack your brain to remember your training when it's someone you love who needs care and you're inwardly panicking.'

Rebecca knew that Hayley had already been through a similar nightmare herself, when her firefighter hero husband had been killed. 'Thank you.'

'We'll give her infant paracetamol for the headache, and then you can take her home,' Hayley said. 'Just check her every hour for the next twenty-four hours. Any worries, bring her straight back.'

Rebecca nodded. 'Will do. And thank you.'

'I'll drop you back at the nursery on the way back to Rebecca's,' Caroline said.

'Thank you. They'll all be so glad to know Jasmine's all right,' Bethany said.

Rebecca called her boss to arrange to take off the next week as unpaid parental leave, then carried Jasmine to her mother's car.

Nathaniel hadn't been looking forward to his afternoon shift, as he knew Rebecca was the one he'd have to call if there were any problems on the labour ward. It would be the first time they'd be in the same room since they'd split up, and it was going to be really awkward. But when he went to the office about a baby whose tocography results concerned him, he saw Tanvir at the desk.

It looked as if Rebecca had changed the rota so she could avoid him. Not that he blamed her.

'Tan, can I ask you to come and check one of my mums? I'm not happy with the baby's heart rate.'

'Sure,' Tanvir said.

'I thought Rebecca was on this afternoon.' The words were out before he could stop them.

'She was. Didn't you hear?'

Nathaniel frowned. 'Hear what?'

'Amara took the call. Jasmine had an accident at nursery and she was brought into the Emergency Department.'

Nathaniel stared at Tanvir in horror. Having

that sort of call would be a nightmare for any parent, but it would be even more of a nightmare for someone in Rebecca's shoes—someone whose husband had died in the Emergency Department after an accident. Rebecca must be worried sick.

'Is Jasmine OK?'

'I don't know,' Tanvir said. 'Though I do know Rebecca's off for the next week on parental leave.'

So it was serious.

Nathaniel's first instinct was to drop everything and go to Rebecca—to be there for her, support her emotionally as well as practically.

And then it hit him.

He loved her.

He loved Jasmine, too, and he wanted to be a family with them. And, even though he'd convinced himself that he wouldn't be enough for Rebecca, he realised that actually he *could* be. From what she'd let slip, he was pretty sure that Lucas would've found excuses to avoid sitting with a sick child or making his wife dinner while she sat with Jasmine; but Nathaniel could do all that.

More than that, he *wanted* to do it. He wanted to be with her. Needed to be with her.

Somehow he got through to the end of his shift—the baby still hadn't made an appearance, but the tocograph showed that his heart-beat was stable and Nathaniel was happy to hand over to the midwife on the next shift.

At the hospital entrance, he stopped at the shop for long enough to buy something for Jasmine and flowers for Rebecca, then headed straight to Rebecca's house.

When the doorbell rang, Rebecca answered the door and was shocked to see Nathaniel standing there.

'Tan told me what happened to Jasmine,' he said in answer to the question that filled her head but wouldn't come out of her mouth. 'How is she?'

'OK,' she answered warily.

'And how are *you*?'

She lifted her chin. 'I'm fine.'

'Are you?' he asked softly. 'You got a call to go to the Emergency Department, for someone you love very much. It must've brought back a lot of tough memories for you.'

It had. 'I'm fine,' she said again.

His expression said that he didn't believe her, but she wasn't going to rely on him for support. He'd made it clear that he didn't want her, and she didn't need his pity.

'I got these for you.' He handed her a gorgeous bunch of flowers.

'Thank you,' she said automatically. She remembered the last time he'd done that—the evening when she'd had a shift that reduced her to tears. When he'd been kind and thoughtful and supportive.

But he'd shown his true colours the day she'd helped deliver his sister's baby. The day he'd dumped her. By *text*. A man who didn't want commitment.

This time, she spoke the question aloud. 'What are you doing here, Nathaniel?'

'I wanted to see you. I was concerned about you and Jasmine.'

Concerned? He hadn't been that concerned about them when he'd sent her that cool, curt text. 'There's no need,' she said stiffly. 'We're fine.'

He huffed out a breath. 'I know I'm an idiot and I did something very, *very* stupid last week. I wouldn't blame you if you never spoke to me again. I know I don't deserve it, but please would you hear me out?'

Part of her wanted to tell him to get lost, but she was too tired to argue. 'Come into the kitchen. Jasmine's asleep in the living room.' Though she was still hurt and angry enough with him not to offer him a drink.

He followed her into the kitchen and she used

the excuse of putting the flowers in water not to look at him.

'I brought Jasmine a present.'

A shiny, glittery pink bag that Rebecca knew her daughter would be instantly attracted to.

'It's a penguin.'

Her favourite animal. He'd clearly remembered that from their day on the river. And she really couldn't work him out. Was Nathaniel Jones a kind, lovely man; or was he a cold-hearted, callous bastard?

'Thank you, but she doesn't need presents.' It was just the sort of thing Lucas had always done, letting her down and then buying her a flashy present to make up for it and promising not to do whatever it was again, when they both knew that of course it would happen again. Presents weren't important. Being there for someone was what really mattered. And Nathaniel had proved to her that he wasn't reliable.

'I'm sorry. What I did was wrong. I didn't mean to hurt you.'

'But you did hurt me,' she said. 'I thought we were getting on fine. We'd dated. I'd met your family. You'd met some of mine. We had *sex*, for pity's sake.'

He flushed. 'Yeah.'

'I don't sleep around, Nathaniel. That night meant something to me.'

'It meant something to me, too.'

'Really? Because, if it did, why did you dump me with no warning?' That wasn't the only thing that rankled. 'And we delivered your sister's baby together. You didn't even tell me how they were.'

'I'm sorry. They're doing brilliantly, really settled into being a family. Delilah's put on weight and Charlotte's blooming.' He grimaced. 'As for your next question—I'm an idiot. A mess. We *were* getting on fine. I was looking forward to meeting your family.'

'So *why* did you dump me?' Hurt made her voice sharp.

'Because I panicked. We'd just delivered Delilah. I looked at Charlotte and Robyn, and I thought about what it must be like to be a new parent, how amazing it must be.'

'And that was your cue to dump me? How?' She shook her head. 'And you didn't even do it in person.'

'I texted you. I know. Which is about the worst way anyone could break off a relationship. I'm so sorry I hurt you.' He took a deep breath. 'I panicked. I thought about how I'd been looking forward to getting married and starting a family—and then the accident happened and I found out the hard way that I wasn't enough for Angela. And then it made me wonder: how could I know that I'd be enough for you?'

That was exactly how she'd felt after her marriage had started to crumble. If Lucas hadn't had the accident, Rebecca knew she wouldn't still be married to him because she hadn't been enough for him. She'd have tried her hardest to make it work, but deep down she knew she wouldn't have been enough.

'You could have talked to me about it,' she said.

'That's exactly what I should've done,' he replied. 'But the more I thought about it, the more I tried to work out what to say, the worse it got and the more I panicked. So I thought the fairest thing to do would be to end it.' He closed his eyes briefly. 'Stupid.'

'Yeah.'

'I was sitting in the waiting room while the midwife was checking them over. Everywhere around me I could see families—everything I wanted. And this voice in my head reminded me that I wasn't enough for Angela—and back then I'd been in a senior role as a site manager. How can I be enough for you now, when I'm only a junior midwife and you're a senior doctor?'

She stared at him. 'You seriously think I'm

that shallow? That I'm worried about how junior or senior you are?'

'No. That's not what I mean. You're not shallow at all.' He took a deep breath. 'I just feel like a fraud. I haven't had a serious relationship since Angie.'

'Because you can't commit.'

'Because I haven't *wanted* to commit,' he said. 'Until you.'

She stared at him. Could she believe him?

'I know it's a big ask,' he said, 'but would you give me a second chance?'

'I come as a package. I can't take chances.' She shook her head. 'I opened my heart to you—I let you into my life, into Jasmine's life—and then you dumped me without any warning. It's like Lucas all over again, happy with the thrill of the chase and then losing interest,' she said. 'And that's not what I want—for me or for Jasmine. What if I give you a second chance and you change your mind and back away from us again?'

'I won't,' he said.

'How can you be so sure?'

'Because,' he said, 'today I heard about Jasmine's accident, and all I wanted to do was to come and find you, be right by your side and support you both through this. It made me realise what an idiot I was being—and that I really want to be a family with you and Jasmine. I love being a godfather, I know I'm going to love being an uncle—and I really, really want to be a dad.'

Something she might not be able to give him. He was worried he wasn't enough for her—but would she be enough for him? It was too important to leave this for later. She had to face the issue. Now.

'Do you mean you want a baby of your own? Because that,' she said, 'might be a problem. I told you about my ectopic pregnancy. What if I have another and lose my other fallopian tube? What if I can't give you children?'

He looked at her, his dark eyes brooding as he thought about it. 'We'll have Jasmine—and I hope in time she'll come to regard me as her dad. I'd never do anything to push Lucas's family out, but I want to be there for Jasmine. And I believe there's more to being a parent than just biology. I want to be your partner and Jasmine's dad. If we're lucky enough to have more children, that'd be wonderful. If not, then we'll still be a family. Just the three of us. Or we could consider fostering or adoption. Families come in all shapes and sizes.'

He wanted to be her partner and Jasmine's dad.

'I want to believe you,' she said. 'I really

want to. But.' Could she really trust him? She couldn't quite bring herself to ask the question, knowing how barbed it was.

'I don't blame you for being wary,' he said. 'You had a rough time with your first marriage, just as I had a rough time with my ex. I find it hard to trust, so I'm guessing you do as well—and I've already let you down once.'

Yes. He had.

'After Angela, I never wanted to get involved with anyone again. And then I met you. I tried to think about you as just a colleague—but everything changed, the moment you kissed me after the abseil. I realised I was falling for you.' He gave her a wry smile. 'You're the first of my girlfriends since the accident who's met my family. And you fitted in, Rebecca. The way you were with them made me think that I'd fit with your family, too.'

'You would,' she admitted. 'Our families are very similar.' And whereas Lucas hadn't had the patience to spend time with her family—or his own—she'd thought Nathaniel was different. A family man. He'd already shown her that, the day they'd spent on the river.

'So give me a chance to prove I won't let you down again.' He paused. 'Just so we're clear on this, you're enough for me.'

'You're trying to tell me you're not Lucas,'

she said. 'In some ways, you're not. You don't have that restlessness and you pay attention. You notice things. You talk to people because you're interested in them, not because you're trying to work the room.' She dragged in a breath. 'But there are some ways where you *are* like Lucas. You're charming. People like you. And if I let myself admit that I love you, I'm scared it's all going to go wrong, just like it did last time. That you'll change. That... That you'll let me down and I'll still be alone but with a broken heart on top of it.'

If I let myself admit that I love you...

The words gave him hope.

She loved him, but she was as scared as he'd been. And no wonder—because he'd already let her down. So now all he could do was tell her exactly what was in his heart. 'I fell in love with you weeks ago. When you were standing on the edge of a building, really scared, but you were going to do it because you'd made a commitment and you don't back down. You see things through.' He waited a beat. 'And so do I. I love you, Rebecca Hart, and I want to be a family with you and Jasmine. I want family afternoons in the park and at the beach and in the garden. I want to bake brownies for school fundraisers. I want to do my share of the nursery run and the sleepless nights and mopping up—just as I want my share of cuddles and home-made cards and bedtime stories. I want family barbecues where your dad and mine spend hours sorting out the music together, and reminiscing, and having a competition to see who can tell the most terrible jokes. And, most of all, I want you. I want to wake up every morning with you in my arms and know that it's going to be a good day because you're the first thing I see.'

He'd opened his heart and told her how he felt. He couldn't do any more. He just had to hope that he would be enough for her.

All he could do now was wait.

Nathaniel loved her.

Rebecca thought about it.

He wanted to be a family with her and Jasmine.

He wanted to wake up with her every morning.

He wanted to take his share of the tough stuff as well as the fun stuff; he was under no illusions that being a parent was easy, and he was prepared to put in the work.

If she let herself believe him, if she trusted him and said yes, she wouldn't be repeating her mistake with Lucas. She could go into this with her eyes wide open. The light-hearted, charming midwife who made the world a brighter place—and who'd still be there when things were difficult. He'd been there when she'd had a rough day and made her feel better. Yes, he'd hurt her, but he regretted it and she really believed he wouldn't do it again. Because she understood now why he'd backed away: she had the same fears for not being enough for someone.

He wasn't sweeping her off her feet; he was standing beside her, an equal partner.

And he'd made it clear that she was what he wanted. That she'd be enough for him. And she knew he was enough for her.

'You love me. You want to be a family with me and Jasmine,' she checked, just to be sure.

'I do.'

His beautiful dark eyes were wary. He'd taken a risk. Trusted her with his heart. And, even though he'd got it wrong, he'd admitted it and taken the blame squarely.

That gave her courage to trust him with her heart, too. 'That's what I want,' she said. 'You. Our family. Everything.' She took a deep breath. 'I love you.'

And it was as if the sun had come out from

behind thick clouds. He stood up and wrapped her in his arms. 'I love you, too. And our family. For ever.'

EPILOGUE

One year later

'READY?' SASKIA MADE a last-minute adjustment to Rebecca's veil. 'Perfect.' She bent down to the two smaller bridesmaids' level; Jasmine and Nathaniel's goddaughter had hit it off from their first meeting and were both thrilled to be bridesmaids. They were even more thrilled that they'd been allowed to choose their dresses, and that they'd chosen the same ones. 'You look lovely, too.'

'So do you, Aunty Sas,' Jasmine said. 'And Mummy looks like a princess.'

'She certainly does. Come on, girls. Let's give her a moment.'

'Are you sure you're ready for this?' Caroline asked.

'I'm sure, Mum.' Rebecca hugged her mother. 'This is going to be the perfect day. Our families, really joined. For ever.'

'You look radiant,' Caroline said. 'And not just bridal radiance.'

'Second trimester radiance,' Rebecca said with a grin. She and Nathaniel had had a few days of worry when they'd realised she'd fallen pregnant, but the early scan had reassured them that it wasn't an ectopic pregnancy, this time round. 'Nathaniel's still finding books to persuade Jas that she won't mind if she ends up with a little brother rather than a sister.'

'The cars are here, Bec!' Saskia called from downstairs.

It felt like the blink of an eye between settling the girls in the car and arriving at the register office. Then finally she was walking down the red carpet towards Nathaniel on her father's arm, Saskia and the girls following her, and Nathaniel's dad singing 'Happy Together' and playing an acoustic guitar.

The room was full to brimming with their closest family and friends. Nathaniel was there waiting for her, his face lit with sheer joy. Rebecca turned round to her bridesmaids and gave them a wink as Mark launched into the chorus of the song, signalling that now was the time to do what they'd been practising for weeks—and then together the bridal party danced and sang their way down the aisle to Nathaniel.

His dark eyes glittered with love and happiness as she drew nearer. All that worrying that they wouldn't be enough for each other: this last year had proved to them both that they were definitely enough. After the accident, Nathaniel had done his share of checking on Jasmine every hour until she'd recovered from her fall, and he'd been there in the park to encourage her to overcome her fears and climb on the bars again, making sure she was safe.

Over the months, Nathaniel had been there for bedtime stories, the school nativity play and Sports Day. He'd been there when Jasmine had woken from a nightmare or been laid low with a bug. And Jasmine had shyly asked him of her own accord if she could call him Daddy.

Leo had adjusted happily to moving from Nathaniel's flat to Rebecca's house, and he spent as much time curled on Rebecca's lap as he did on Nathaniel's.

Nathaniel bought flowers with Jasmine for Rebecca every Friday evening and made her mugs of tea exactly how she liked them; Rebecca had learned from Jason's mum how to cook Nathaniel's favourite dishes, and she'd become close to his sister and parents.

Their lonely struggles had turned into a warm, close, loving family—for both of them.

As she reached him in front of the registrar,

Nathaniel greeted her with a kiss. 'My beautiful bride. My for ever family. I love you,' he said.

'I love you, too,' she replied, and the registrar began the service.

* * * * *

*If you enjoyed this story, check out
these other great reads from
Kate Hardy*

Fling with Her Hot-Shot Consultant
Mistletoe Proposal on the Children's Ward
A Nurse and a Pup to Heal Him
Heart Surgeon, Prince…Husband!

All available now!